7 Ways
To Manage Pain
With CBD

7 Ways
To Manage Pain
With CBD

THE TOTAL NEWBIES GUIDE TO UNDERSTANDING
CBD BASICS, COMBATING PAIN USING IT IN
MULTIPLE FORMS, & FINDING A BETTER QUALITY
OF LIFE APART FROM OPIOID USE.

DAVID ANTHONY SCHROEDER

Marketing by: CannaWeb Solutions
A 21st. Century Digital Marketing Agency
https://cannawebsolutions.com

7 Ways To Manage Pain With CBD

Contact Information:
Website: https://thecbdwriter.com
Customer Service: custserv@thecbdwriter.com
Sales: sales@thecbdwriter.com
General Help and Information: inforequest@thecbdwriter.com
Advertising: advertising@thecbdwriter.com
Public Relations: prdept@thecbdwriter.com

Publisher's Note

We have done our best to carefully research and compile this manual only from a source believed to be authentic and reliable. However we cannot guarantee total accuracy or completeness.

If you would be kind enough to bring to our attention any errors you may find, we will include your corrections in our next edition. We will also send you a complimentary bonus manual as a token of our appreciation.

If you feel we've missed something and should include it in this book, let us know. If we use it, we'll send you a free updated copy of the book for taking the effort.

Email: inforequest@thecbdwriter.com
Website: https://thecbdwriter.com

DEDICATION

To the billions of human beings on
this planet, whether black, white, brown, yellow, red,
or purple with pink polka dots, who are part of the only race
that has ever been known to mankind, the human race:

To the brave men and women who have gone before me and have
gallantly fought and given their lives for my freedom, and to the men
and women who have fought and continue to fight for my freedom
today, and to those men and women retired from the Battlefield:

To those who put their lives on the line daily, our first responders,
whether fire, bullets, emergency, disaster, life, or death,
you put others before yourselves to save lives:

And to those who live with constant
physical pain daily:

I dedicate this
book to
you

.

FOREWORD

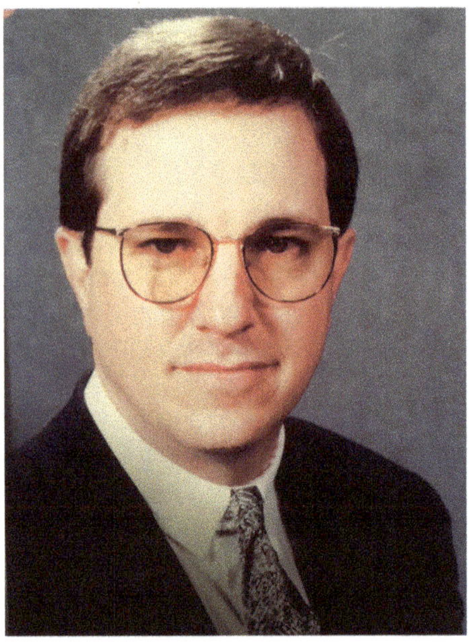

Dr. David Allen, M.D.

I'm very pleased to have been asked by David Anthony Schroeder to give a foreword to his wonderfully written book. We are the pioneers of this new science called the Endocannabinoid Signaling System. It is a regulatory system of all human and animal cells that regulates homeostasis or the ability to stay alive in ever-changing cellular environments.

This is the only science that has been restricted by law! This science is mostly UNKNOWN to our current medical education system. Your own physician probably has no clue of its existence. (See my article entitled "Ignorance is Not Bliss" in Cannabis Digest) https://bit.ly/not-bliss

I am famous for my statement; "The discovery of the Endocannabinoid signaling system is the single most important scientific study in human history and will save more lives than the discovery and application of sterile surgical technique. This means more people will be saved by manipulation of the ECS than are currently saved by sterile surgical procedures!"

Since you can eat cannabis raw in an unheated form, you can enjoy its benefits, and it won't get you high (cause euphoria). Cannabis has "unheard of" "unrivaled medical benefits!" This makes cannabis a Nutraceutical and metabolic necessity. If your ECS is not functioning properly, it brings you closer to death!

The ECS functions by cannabinoid receptors that are actually protein chains embedded in all cell membranes. These protein receptors act like antenna that react when certain chemicals float by and attach themselves to the CB1 receptors. These receptors or antenna act like a lock and key with the chemicals they are designed to couple with.

Most people are familiar with insulin attaching to insulin receptors and causing glucose to go from the blood into the cell. So only insulin attaches to insulin receptors, and only cannabinoids attach to cannabinoid receptors. When cannabinoids from the plant or from your own body (endogenous or Endocannabinoids) bind on to CB1 or CB2 receptors, it regulates cellular metabolism to keep you alive.

Every metabolic function that you can think of oscillates between a high and low point. So, for instance, your pH will go up and down, your glucose levels go up and down, your Testosterone and estrogen go up and down. All physiological processes go up and down. If they go too high or too low, they are incompatible with life, and you die. Life (homeostasis) is in the middle ground between the highs and lows.

All humans and animals have an ECS or Endocannabinoid regulatory system. Some humans have a proper functioning Endocannabinoid system and would be considered Endocannabinoid endowed. Others whose endocannabinoid system is dysfunctional would be considered Endocannabinoid deficient. This makes cannabis a superfood and is Essential for life and proper metabolism. A super vitamin!

This book is teaching a new science that is not even taught to our medical doctors. Dr. Allen's "ignorance is not bliss" study proved only 13% of American Medical Schools even mention this science, and not one medical school in the United States teaches the science behind cannabis as medicine!

We are in the infancy of this science that this book is revealing. We are the pioneers!

My first day of surgical residency, my chief resident spoke to the new residents and said two important things!

1. If we want your opinion we will tell it to you,
2. The pioneers get the arrows!

David B. Allen M.D.

cali215doc@gmail.com
https://bit.ly/not-bliss

TABLE OF CONTENTS

" **A HOSPITAL BED IS A PARKED TAXI WITH THE METER RUNNING.** "

Groucho Marx.

Introduction

My Dear Friend,

Thank you for getting this book, 7 ways to manage pain with CBD. My biggest hope is that this book will give you one or more ways to manage your pain whether joint, muscle, chronic, or other, using CBD and relying much less on doctor prescribed narcotics.

"Primum Non Nocere."
This is the classical Latin phrase that
means "first, to do no harm."

When a person becomes the student, and the "student" becomes the doctor, he or she takes the Hippocratic Oath - the doctor must, and I emphasize this person, no longer the student must have two very special objectives in his purview with regards to healing the human body, namely, "to do good or to do no harm." (Hippocrates)

What is the state of today's medical community?

Let's Turn on the TV

The commercial tells you your knee pain can be kept to a minimum if you take Super XYZ drug, see your doctor and ask for Super XYZ. Oh and by the way, some people who took Super XYZ experienced diarrhea, fatigue, anemia, vomiting, headaches, depression, and destruction to their liver. 68 out of 102 people lost their eye sight, and others had thoughts of committing suicide. Ask your doctor and see if Super XYZ is right for your knee pain.

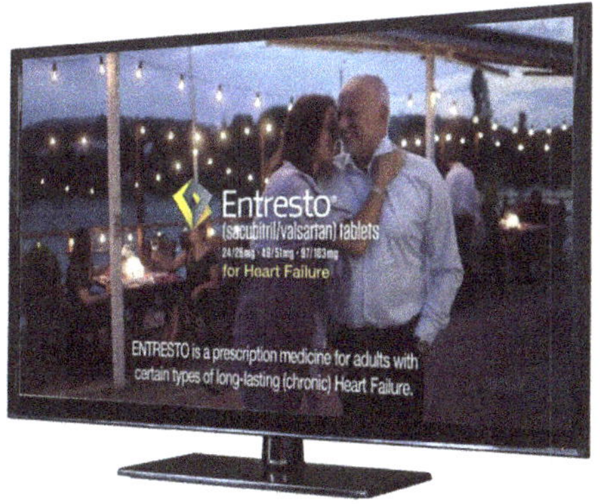

You, being so moved by the content of the TV commercial go and see your doctor, you tell him you have knee pain, and you want Super XYZ. Well, it just so happens that Pharmaceutical Drug Maker, "Give Me All Your Money Inc." has put together a program for doctors in their particular field or specialty.

Doctors Get To Cash In

Now in the 21st century, Dr. Heal Me Goode, can be hired by the pharmaceutical company "Give Me All Your Money Inc." and receive remuneration while prescribing you the drug Super XYZ for your pain ailments.

Here's how it works; first, Dr. Heal Me Goode gets paid by your insurance company, your deductibles, and your co-payments. Good so far, but doctors that write large amounts of prescriptions get compensated in a variety of ways including travel, meals, consulting, speaking fees, and royalties.

Chicago Tribune August 17th. 2017 "More than 28,000 Illinois doctors accepted $74.1 million from pharmaceutical and medical device companies in 2016, excluding payments for research, according to a Tribune analysis of recently released federal data." See endnotes page for additional information.

The Pharmaceutical Company's Stand to Lose Billions of Dollars Because of CBD.

What on earth is going on? What about you, the patient? What happened to "Do No Harm"? Let me sum it up: Heal Me Goode gets rewarded, (some, rewarded handsomely) from "Give Me All Your Money Inc.'s" drug marketing program, he's given limited time to resolve your complaint and to get paid from "We Got You Covered Insurance Company," and you... you get narcotics that temporarily relieve pain but cause more damage and produce side-effects worse than the actual infirmity. Ah "Houston, we have a problem." See Footnotes page for additional information.

Pain and what is it?

Pain, what is it, how do we deal with it, how do we get over it, how do we get healed from it? That's the question you ask yourself every day, and the answer is always the same. Another day of pain, another day of narcotics, another day of disgust from how they make you feel and what they do to you physically.

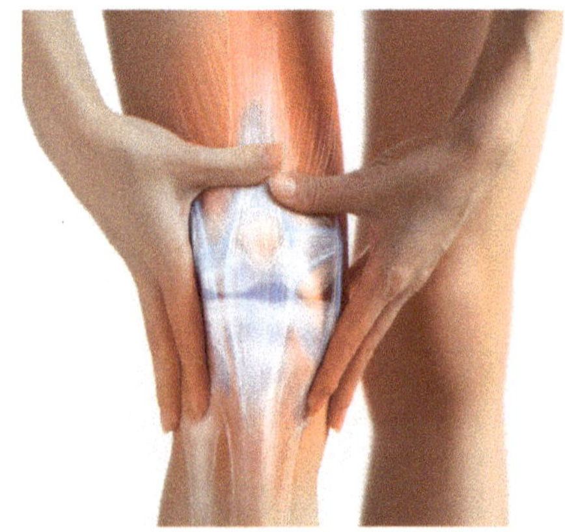

I'm not a doctor so I cannot give you the medical description of pain. But I have dealt with pain off and on all of my life, in various places throughout my body, and now that I'm over 50, I am all the more aware of the pain just from the aging perspective.

I can describe pain in a certain way that might be Universal enough for you to understand, but there are better descriptions.

Here is pain as broken down and defined by WebMD:

Acute Pain and Chronic Pain

There are several ways to categorize pain. One is to separate it into acute pain and chronic pain. Acute pain typically comes on suddenly and has a limited duration. It's frequently caused by damage to tissue such as bone, muscle, or organs, and the onset is often accompanied by anxiety or emotional distress. Chronic pain lasts longer than acute pain and is generally somewhat resistant to medical treatment. It's usually associated with a long-term illness, such as osteoarthritis. In some cases, such as with fibromyalgia, it's one of the defining characteristics of the disease. Chronic pain can be the result of damaged tissue, but very often is attributable to nerve damage. Both acute and chronic pain can be debilitating, and both can affect and be affected by a person's state of mind. But the nature of chronic pain -- the fact that it's ongoing and in some cases seems almost constant -- makes the person who has it more susceptible to psychological consequences such as depression and anxiety. At the same time, psychological distress can amplify the pain.

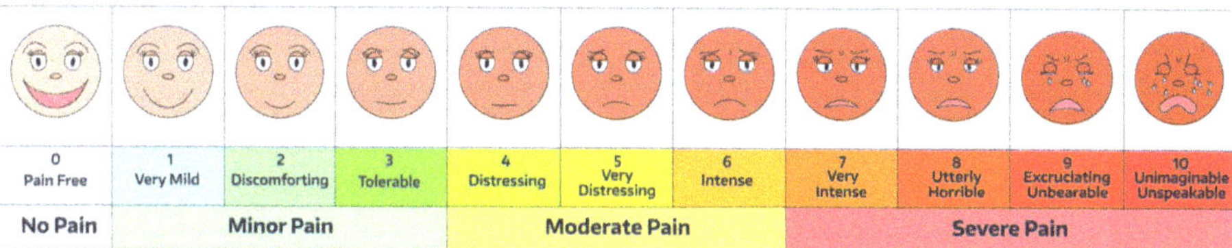

Feeling perfectly normal	Nagging, annoying, but doesn't interfere with most daily activities. Patient able to adapt to pain psychologically and with medication or devices such as cushions.	Interferes significantly with daily living activities. Requires lifestyle changes but patient remains independent. Patient unable to adapt to pain.	Disabling; unable to perform living activities. Unable to engage in normal activities. Patient is disabled and unable to function independently.

The Center for Disease Control released a study in September of 2018 stating that they estimate 50 Million Americans live in chronic pain. In years past, some clinical studies said as much as 110 Million Americans are living in chronic pain. Can you imagine how much money has been paid to big pharmaceutical companies to create and sell pain management narcotics? BILLIONS!!!!!

Can you imagine the damage that has been done to our body's from those incredibly dangerous and harmful chemicals called drugs? This book is the layman's guide to finding appropriate applications for using CBD that work for you.

LET'S SEE WHAT SOME DOCTORS WILLING TO SPEAK OUT HAVE BEEN QUOTED AS SAYING ABOUT USING CBD

Dr. David Allen, M.D.

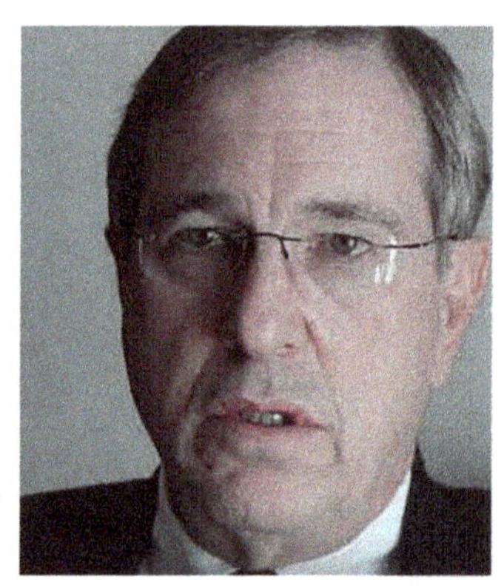

A retired cardiac surgeon and a member of the International Cannabinoid Research Society (ICRS), a cannabinoid research scientist.

"Basically the endocannabinoid system is responsible for homeostasis. Most people don't understand what that really means but it's the body's ability to maintain itself and function in a proper environment. So it's critically important that doctors in the future understand this control mechanism.

We're finding out that manipulation of this endocannabinoid system will control diabetes, it controls cancer, it controls whether you can survive a heart attack or a stroke. So this is critically important for doctors to understand this new science.

The discovery of the endocannabinoid system is the single most important medical scientific discovery ever and will save more lives than the discovery and application of sterile surgical technique. I'm a heart surgeon saying that. So more people will be saved by manipulation of the endocannabinoid system then are currently saved by surgery."

"Cannabis is remarkably safe. Although not harmless, it is surely less toxic than most of the conventional medicine it could replace if it were legally available. Cannabis has never caused an overdose death." - Lester Grinspoon, M.D.

Dr. Rob Streisfeld, NMD

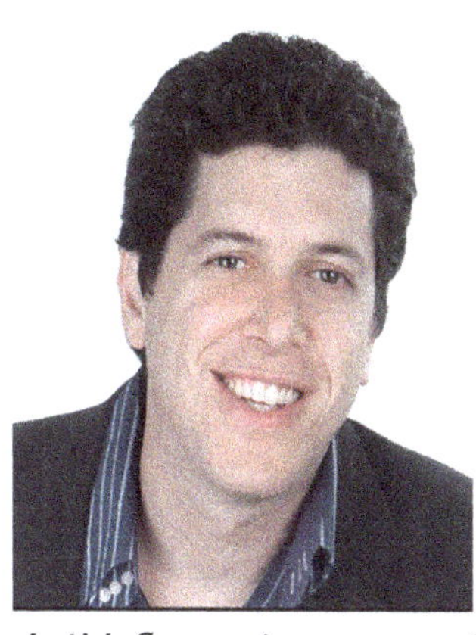

"Working in both Preventative Medicine and in the Natural Products/Dietary Supplement Industries for almost 20 years, I have seen several new ingredients, compounds, and herbs touted as the next "big thing".

Cannabis, and its over 500 compounds offer an amazing opportunity to promote health and manage disease. Cannabidiol, or CBD, seems to offer the most widespread usage, and is likely the single ingredient or plant compound most being researched around the world today.

Anti-inflammatory properties, neuro-protective benefits, immune support and anti-oxidant properties are all found with CBD.... With the potential for innovation in drug development, as well as wellness products for everyday consumers, CBD holds tremendous value to support/optimize a person's health and shift society's perception to accept the healing power of this plant and others.

CBD has been especially well received as it doesn't have the psychoactive effects that THC has. People of all ages (and their pets) are getting benefits in a safe, non-toxic way when using Cannabis and its compounds."

- 'On The Record' Quote

Doctor Alan Shackelford

A Harvard trained physician. He's also among a handful of doctors in Colorado who give prescriptions for medical marijuana.

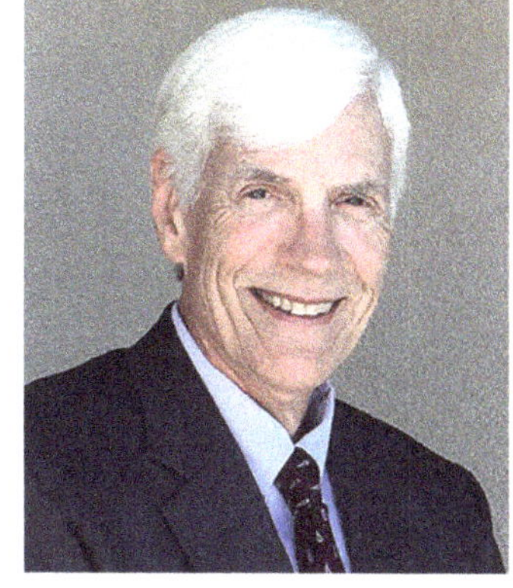

From the moment Charlotte entered his office he knew she was in trouble. While he was just examining her she had two seizures.

Doctor Alan Shackelford: "She failed everything. There were no more options for her. Everything had been tried,… except cannabis."

Here's how scientists think it might work.

Marijuana is made up of two ingredients THC – that's the psychoactive part that makes you high. And CBD also called Cannabidiol. It's the CBD that scientists think modulate electrical and chemical activity to help quiet the excessive activity in the brain that causes seizures.

Daniel Clauw, MD

Professor of anesthesiology at the University of Michigan

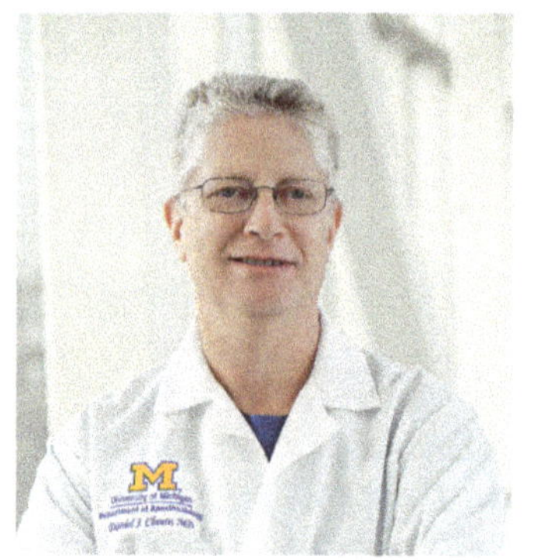

Daniel Clauw believes that CBD may have real benefits for people living with chronic pain. He cites a recent clinical trial from pharmaceutical company Zynerba (for which Dr. Clauw has consulted) that found that a CBD-derived topical drug provided pain relief to patients suffering from knee osteoarthritis.

He says he wants pain patients to know that CBD products may be worth a try—and that they may provide relief, even without the high that products with THC produce.

"I don't think we have that many good drugs for pain, and we know that CBD has fewer side effects than opioids or even nonsteroidal anti-inflammatory drugs, which can cause bleeding and cardiovascular problems," he says. "If I have an elderly patient with arthritis and a little bit of CBD can make their knees feel better, I'd prefer they take that than some other drugs."

"A systematic review of 18 randomized controlled trials (RCTs) with a total of 766 participants with chronic non-cancer pain found that 15/18 trials showed a significant analgesic effect of cannabinoids, compared to placebo."

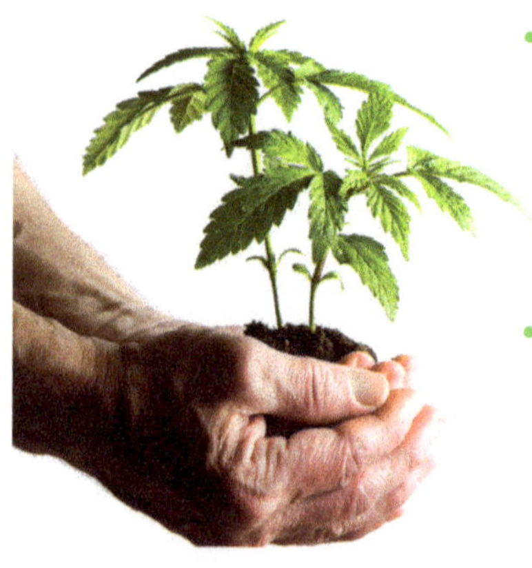

- *Conditions studied included neuropathic pain, "chronic pain", rheumatoid arthritis, fibromyalgia, and central pain in multiple sclerosis.*

- *No serious adverse events were reported.* - British Journal of Clinical Pharmacology: "Cannabinoids for treatment of chronic non-cancer pain; a systematic review of randomized trials"

THE GREATEST EVIL IS PHYSICAL PAIN.

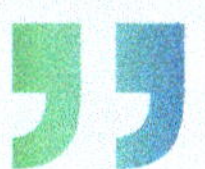

Saint Augustine

CHAPTER ONE

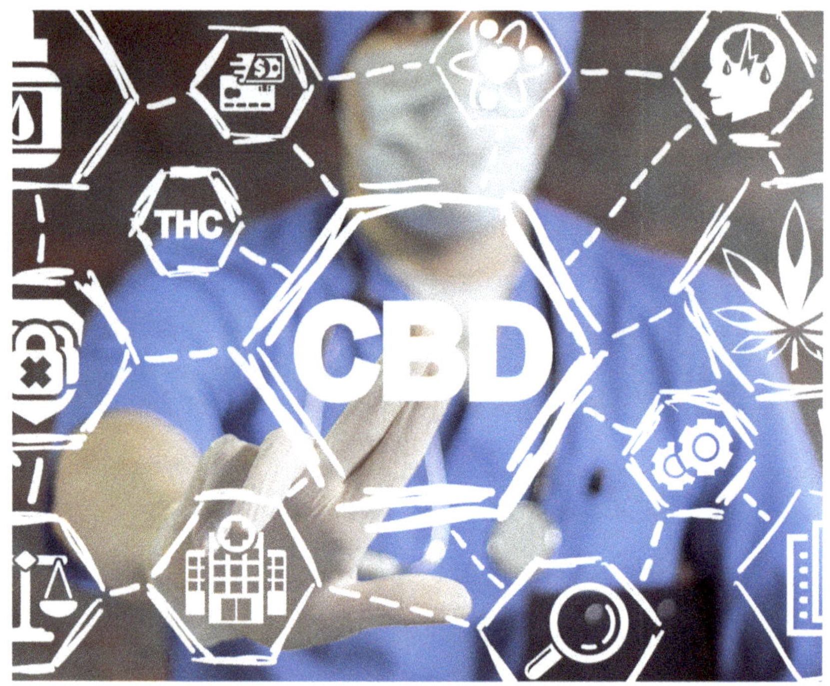

What is CBD?

What is CBD?

Cannabidiol

CBD is one of many cannabinoids found in the hemp plant. Most products on the market are actually hemp extracts containing a broad spectrum of ingredients, such as vitamin E, coconut, chlorophyll, terpenes and somewhere in the area of 50 to over 100 other cannabinoids, including CBD.

By definition, CBD is short for cannabidiol, a compound that is extracted from the hemp plant.

Note: Some CBD oil products may contain very low levels of THC, the compound in cannabis that produces a "high" – but having it doesn't mean you're getting high.

The claims of health and wellness benefits stretch as far as the left is from the right, but in this book, we will cover the areas dealing with pain relief that include medical research to back it up. You'll find links to lots of studies in the appendix.

What determines the difference between Cannabis and Hemp is the level of THC in the plant. The cannabis plant high in THC is also known by its slang name, marijuana, but we will use the correct term, cannabis. Hemp is the high CBD plant, and that is the plant that we are focused on.

Think of it this way, one plant, two species. Hemp (No get high) and Cannabis (Get you high).

HEMP CBD VS. CANNABIS CBD

- Non-psychoactive
- Does not result in feelings of euphoria
- Does not cause intoxication
- CBD contains trace amounts of THC only about 0.3%

- Associated with the feeling of being high
- Results in euphoria and psychoactivity
- Cannabis contains about 5-10% THC
- Illegal in most states without a Medical Marijuana Card

Today I think most people are seeking alternatives to addictive pharmaceutical opioids with harsh side effects. They want medicine that is more in tune with their body's natural cycle. By tapping into how we function biologically on a molecular level, CBD can provide us with relief for most pain and also inflammation.

A WORD ABOUT FULL SPECTRUM CBD–VS–CBD ISOLATE

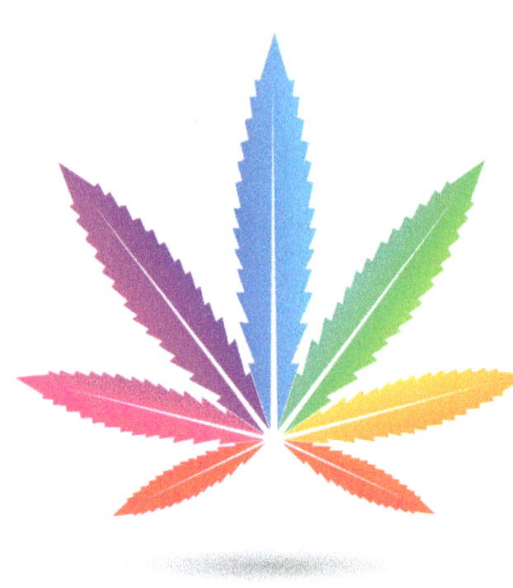

Some manufacturer labels will make the distinction or point out that their CBD is either full spectrum or whole plant CBD.

Full spectrum or whole plant means that the product contains other cannabinoids. It also means that that product could also include or contain trace amounts (0.3% or less) of THC, along with cannabinol (CBN) and tetrahydrocannabivarin (THCV). This includes other cannabinoids such as CBL, and CBCVA, plus some manufacturers may incorporate scented or sweet-smelling cannabis terpenes such as pinene, terpinolene, ocimene, and limonene. See the Terpenes list page 57.

Some clinical researchers have found that full spectrum CBD may be more potent due to its synergistic reactions with the terpenes and minor cannabinoids present. Also, keep in mind that trace amounts of THC in full spectrum CBD products COULD and I mean COULD compromise a drug test.

If the label states that it is CBD only then you know what you are not getting. Everything else, CBD alone. It's essential that you read the labels and understand what is in the product that you want to use. There is more about reading labels in chapter 3.

Why is CBD being considered as the Miracle BreakThrough

For starters, there is extensive scientific research with the most prominent portion being completed by the Israelis over the last 50 years and another big portion sponsored by our own U.S. government, and secondly, there are a plethora of anecdotal accounts from patients and physicians highlighting CBD's potential for treating a wide range of maladies, including (but not limited to):

- Autoimmune diseases (Such as inflammation and rheumatoid arthritis)
- Neurological conditions (Such as Alzheimer's, Dementia, Epilepsy, Multiple Sclerosis, Parkinson's, Strokes, and Traumatic Brain Injuries would be included in that)
- Metabolic syndromes (Such as Diabetes and Obesity)
- Neuropsychiatric illness (Such as Autism, ADHD, PTSD, and Alcoholism)
- Gut disorders (Such as Colitis and Crohn's disease)
- Cardiovascular dysfunction (Such as Atherosclerosis and Arrhythmia)
- Skin diseases (Such as Acne, Dermatitis, and Psoriasis)

"Dear Honorable Jeff Sessions,

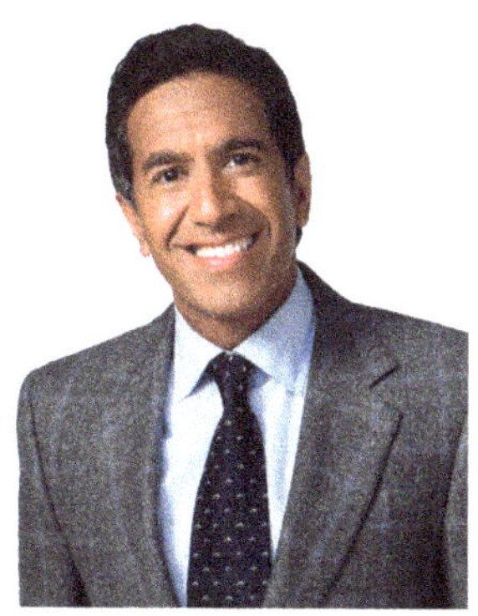

I feel obligated to share the results of my five-year-long investigation into the medical benefits of the cannabis plant. Before I started this worldwide, in-depth investigation, I was not particularly impressed by the results of medical marijuana research, but a few years later, as I started to dedicate time with patients and scientists in various countries, I came to a different conclusion.

The consensus is clear: Cannabis can effectively treat pain. The National Academies of Sciences, Engineering, and Medicine arrived at this conclusion last year after what it described as the "most comprehensive studies of recent research" on the health effects of cannabis. - Dr. Sanjay Gupta

Open letter to Attorney Jeff Sessions regarding cannabis.

HOW DOES IT WORK?

QUICK OVERVIEW OF THE ENDOCANNABINOID SYSTEM

The Human Endocannabinoid System

CBD, CBN, and THC fit like a lock and key into existing human receptors. These receptors are part of the endocannabinoid system which impact physiological processes affecting pain modulation, memory, and appetite plus anti-inflammatory effects and other immune system responses. The endocannabinoid system compromises two types of receptors, CB1 and CB2, which serve distinct functions in human health and well-being.

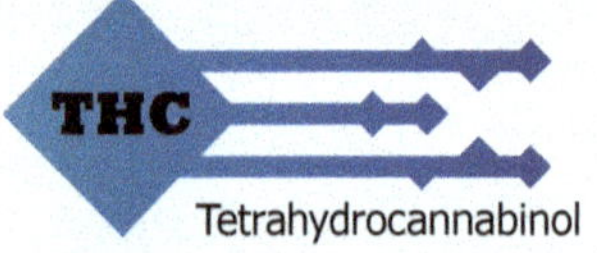

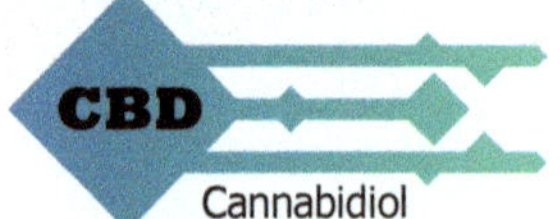

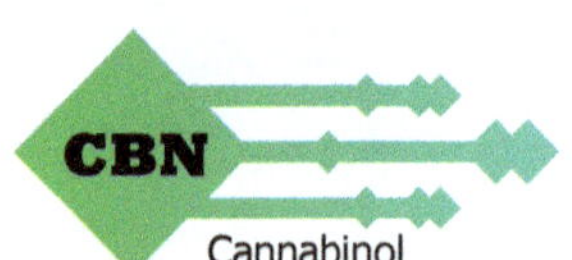

CB1 receptors are primarily found in the brain and central nervous system, and to a lesser extent in other tissues.

CBD does not directly "fit" CB1 or CB2 receptors but has powerful indirect effects still being studied.

CB2 receptors are mostly in the perepheral organs, especially cells associated with the immune system.

This illustration is what we've learned over the last 30 years of discovering the ECS. This is the best explanation I've found in 40 years of using the whole cannabis plant for my own issues.

Hemp cannabinoid extract affects the endocannabinoid system by activating what are called the CB1 and CB2 receptors located throughout your body. The endocannabinoid system (ECS) regulates the proper function of a wide range of your body's processes. The main mechanisms of the endocannabinoid system modulate pleasure, energy, well being, and helps support the body back to health when injured or fighting off disease.

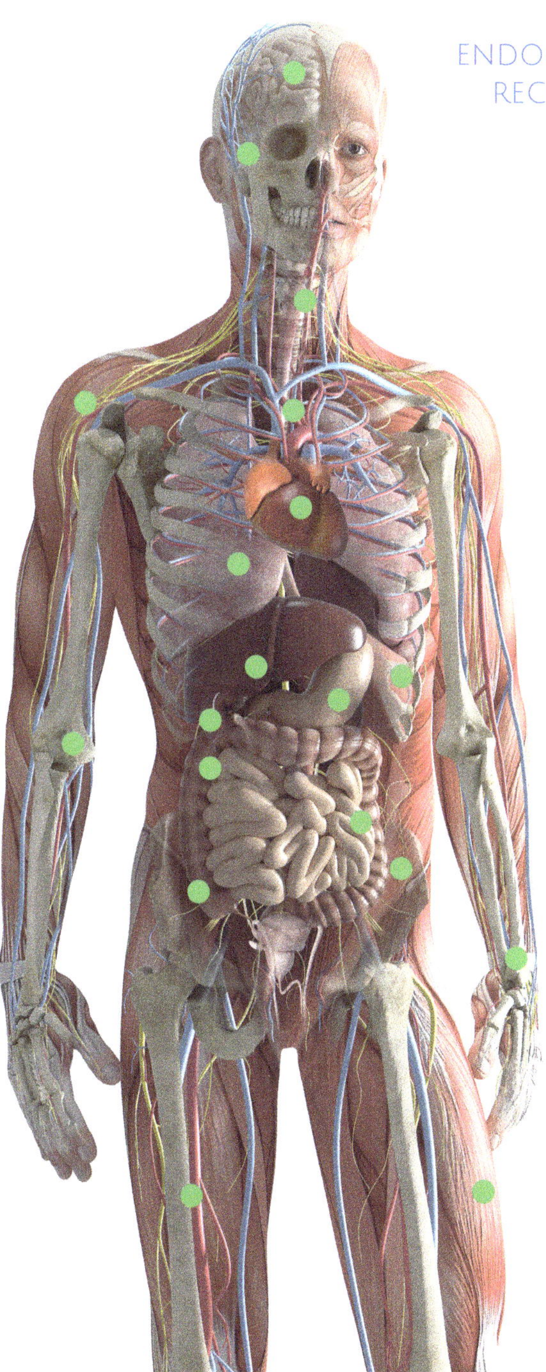

WHERE THE ENDOCANNABINOID SYSTEM RECEPTORS ARE FOUND IN THE BODY

- nervous system
- immune system
- digestive system
- endocrine glands
- brain
- heart
- lungs
- kidneys
- liver
- spleen
- bones
- muscles
- blood vessels
- lymph cells and fat cells

To give you the best explanation for simple understanding, I'm going to let the authors from ProjectCBD.org explain how CBD works:

"CBD and THC interact with our bodies in a variety of ways. One of the main ways they impact us is by mimicking and augmenting the effects of the compounds in our bodies called "endogenous cannabinoids" - so named because of their similarity to the compounds found in the cannabis plant. These "endocannabinoids" are part of a regulatory system called the "endocannabinoid system".

"The discovery of the endocannabinoid system has significantly advanced our understanding of health and disease. It has major implications for nearly every area of medical science and helps to explain how and why CBD and THC are such versatile compounds – and why cannabis is such a widely consumed mood-altering plant, despite its illegal status."

"The endocannabinoid system plays a crucial role in regulating a broad range of physiological processes that affect our everyday experience – our mood, our energy level, our intestinal fortitude, immune activity, blood pressure, bone density, glucose metabolism, how we experience pain, stress, hunger, and more."

What happens if the endocannabinoid system doesn't function properly? What are the consequences of a chronically deficient or overactive endocannabinoid system?

In a word, **disease.**

"Cutting-edge science has shown that the endocannabinoid system is dysregulated in nearly all pathological conditions.

Thus, it stands to reason that "modulating endocannabinoid system activity may have therapeutic potential in almost all diseases affecting humans," as Pal Pacher and George Kunos, scientists with the U.S. National Institutes of Health (NIH), suggested in a 2014 publication."

"By modulating the endocannabinoid system and enhancing endocannabinoid tone, CBD and THC can slow – or in some cases stop – disease progression." (CBD 101 - Project CBD)

Visualizing The ECS

Think of the endocannabinoid system as a car. A car is made up of various systems. Such as:

- the cooling system
- the sound system
- the heating, and air system
- the ignition system
- the braking system, etc.

For the last thirty years, cars have come off the line with a computer system. That computer system is attached to sensors located throughout the vehicle. You find them in the engine, the gas tank, the wheels, the exhaust, the brakes, and elsewhere. Sensors alert you when there is a possible problem.

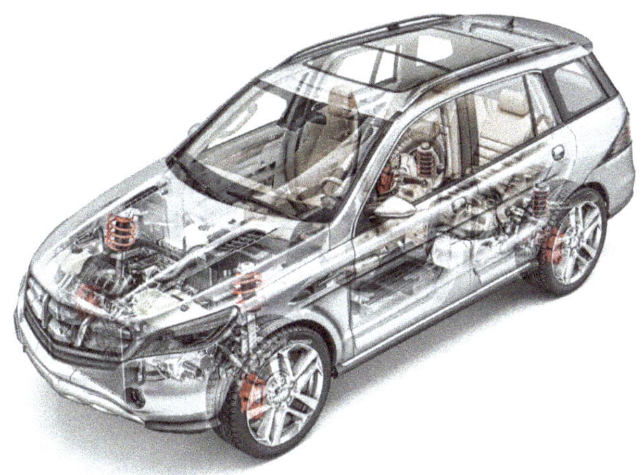

There is one thing that ties everything together; it's called the wiring harness. The wiring harness connects the ignition switch to the battery, to the computer, to its sensors, to run the engine. You drive until your tire sensors tell you, you have low air pressure or that it's time for an oil change. Each system has a purpose and a function; this way, each part of the car operates without failure.

The endocannabinoid system is like that wiring harness. It connects your brain (the computer) to your heart (the battery). It then connects to the rest of your body, the limbs, the internal organs, the body's largest organ, the epidermis, and its sensors, cannabinoid (CB1 & CB2) receptors. The ECS ties everything together, and signals back to the brain similar to sensors on your car. Then the brain releases its chemicals as the body needs.

SIDE EFFECTS

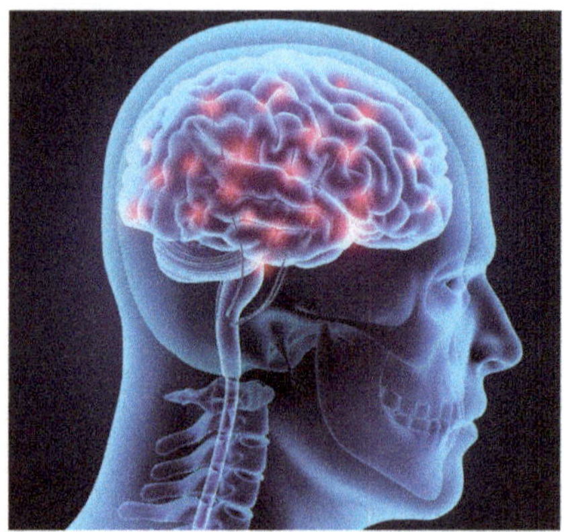

A Bit About CBD Side Effects

There are not many side effects that are associated with CBD (in any form), not like you hear on commercials. One of the more commonly reported issues is a tendency to experience some dry mouth after taking CBD.

There have been some reported instances of starting out with too much and users experiencing some drowsiness.

In a world full of opioid treatments with a long list of adverse side effects — most of which are worse than what you have — a bit of dry mouth or drowsiness, something that is temporary and doesn't have a destructive effect on you I think is perfectly acceptable for a decrease in pain-related symptoms.

Talk To Your Doctor

A BIG side effect for people on prescribed medications: CBD can decrease your liver's ability to process other drugs. If you're doctor prescribed heart medication and you start ingesting CBD, you could be doing more harm than good. Talk to your physician first in these instances about CBD. In some cases, it may not be the right time for you start.

I should point out that if you are only using topicals to manage your pain, then chances are extremely high that you'll experience none of these side effects. The reason being when putting on the skin, the delivery system to the bloodstream is prolonged.

Can You Overdose On CBD?

The truth is it is next to impossible to overdose on CBD. If you're using it sensibly and according to the labels instructions you won't have any problems.

Some users who take too much CBD will have some drowsiness. But I have to admit, sleeping may not even be considered a harmful side-effect if you suffer from insomnia.

Always use caution and read the labels for instructions on the proper amount to use.

IS CBD INTOXICATING?

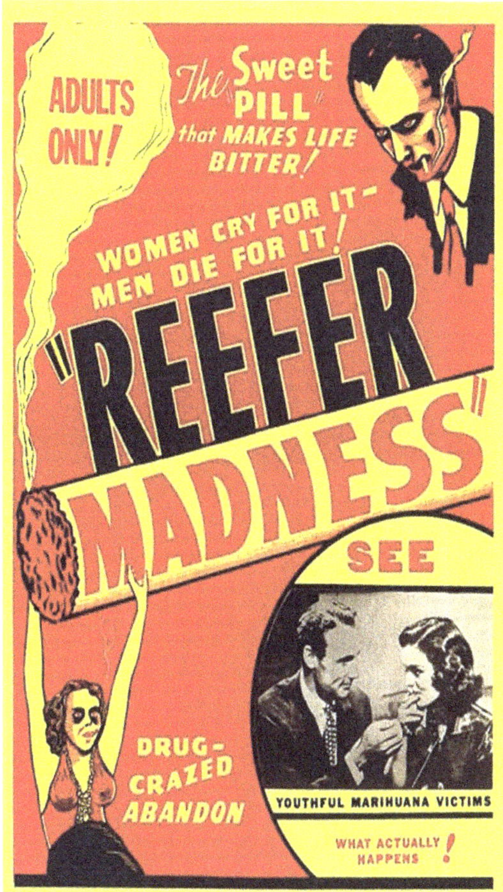

It's true, Hemp CBD products are federally legal and can be shipped over state lines. So you may ask yourself, "Can Hemp CBD get me high?" In a word no. CBD alone cannot get you high.

CBD is high in quantity in the hemp plant while THC is high in quantity in the cannabis plant. Hemp does contain minute amounts of THC, but as long as the hemp oil product has less than 0.3%, it is a safe source for cannabinoid consumption.

Not only will CBD not get you high, but it actually counteracts the high effects of THC, the compound that gets you high. Think of it as Yin & Yang. One balances out the other.

Use a high-quality Hemp CBD product that contains no THC for your pain needs, and you should be fine in the products you choose. Or at least for shipping across state lines.

"CBD was to help sooth my anxiety. It was a huge relief for me to feel like myself, yet the edge was gone. The bonus of the whole thing was the relief from aches and pains. It immediately alleviated 90% of my pain."

\- Tom Hanks (Actor)

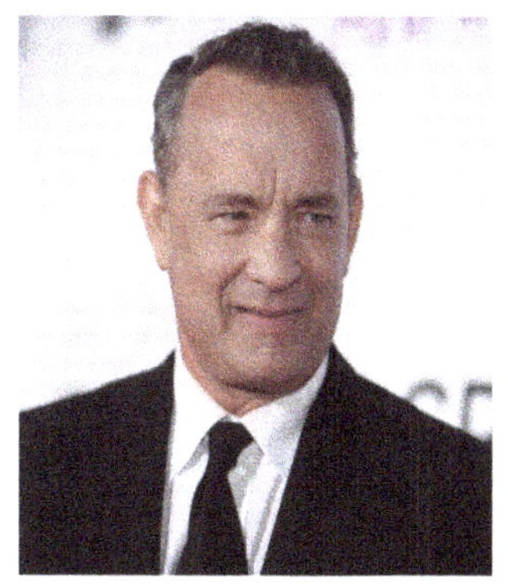

7 Ways to Manage Pain with CBD

THE BIG QUESTION:

WHAT IF

IT DOESN'T WORK FOR ME?

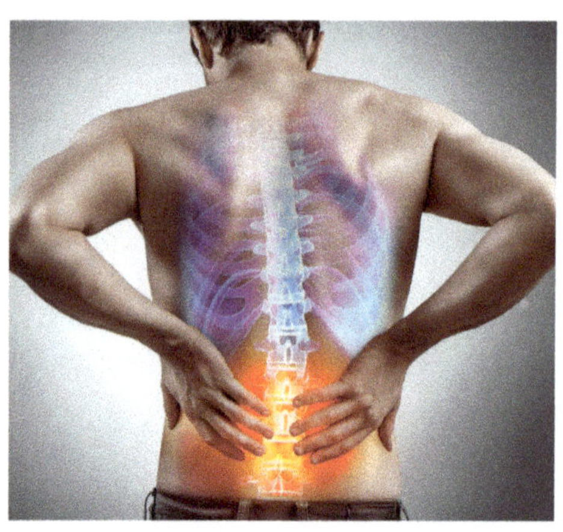

OK, so maybe you have tried CBD and said, "naa, this doesn't work."

Well, the first thing I think is what was the quality of the CBD product that you used or ingested. Laboratories that test cannabis and hemp products find that many manufacturers have as little as 2% CBD per serving in their oil or product, but make big claims on the label.

That my friend is a very low-quality product and I would not expect you to get any benefit from that. In fact, I would expect you to be turned off from CBD and never consider it again. I wouldn't blame you. Please see chapters 3 and 4 on reading labels and lab test results. They'll give you a good understanding of buying a better product.

Bad product does nothing for you. It makes money for the snake-oil salesman who sold it to you. Don't purchase with haste. Use the checklist in the appendix to avoid poor quality CBD products.

The second reason why it might not have given you any relief is that the amount used may not have been enough. Many factors affect the amount you need to feel relief. Read chapter 2 regarding dosing and find the right amount of CBD for your physical needs. Remember, always start small and slow. You want to make sure you don't have any adverse reactions to CBD. Then work your way up to where you feel relief. Don't give up, at least not too soon. Don't be afraid of taking 40mg or 50mg if that is the amount you need. CBD is not a "one size fits all."

The third possible reason is old, CBD oil. Generally, oils go rancid over time. In the 1800s, medical cannabis tinctures and compounds that were consumed came in very dark-colored bottles because the light exposure would decrease the longevity of the cannabis product, thus rendering it useless after long periods of light. If you purchased an old product, or if you've had it for more than a year, it more than likely wouldn't work.

If you've passed that date, don't use the product. If it tastes funny, don't use it. If you just purchased it, ask for your money back.

A fourth reason CBD may not have helped you is that it needs to be taken regularly for more than two or three days at a time. "The most effective neuropathic pain relief occurs after 1 week of daily CBD treatment," says senior author Gabriella Gobbi, MD, PhD, professor of psychiatry, Neurobiological Psychiatry Unit, McGill University, Montreal, Canada.

I want you to see this picture of a General overlooking his battlefield. He observes the battle is fiercest on his west flank, and his enemy is overpowering his army. He sends a

"You Can Beat The Conman at His Own Game With The CBD Buying Checklist in The Appendix."

regiment of soldiers to protect his territory to stop the enemy from breaking through.

During the battle, some are killed, some are wounded, some run out of ammunition, and sadly some defect. Fortunately, the next day, there are more soldiers on his west flank than he had the previous day. Again he sends another regiment. Some are killed, some are wounded, some run out of ammunition, and some defect.

Each day the Generals army fighting at the west flank grows and gets stronger as he keeps sending in fresh troops. Finally, the general turns the tide to his favor, and now the enemy is on the run.

Every new day that you take CBD, you're sending in fresh troops on to your personal battlefield. If today is day one, then by the consumption method that you've chosen, those are your soldiers. CBD does wear off. It's only temporary relief. During the battle, some are killed, some are wounded, some run out of ammunition, and sadly some defect.

Acute pain from injuries like car accidents, expect to use a consistent daily dosage amount maybe even several times throughout the day for at least six to eight weeks and maybe longer if needed. For chronic pain users, your game plan is the same, but to wage war on multiple fronts. CBD can be swallowed or used sublingually, taken via the rectum or vagina, inhaled via plant or vape form, and can be applied topically. But it has to become apart of your lifestyle just like coffee, sugar, or Redbull.

Reason five is having a high tolerance to other drugs and alcohol. If you have a history of using other drugs, such as pain killers, or using alcohol, here is my caution to you. Don't be surprised if you don't feel anything. If that's you, then the chances are that you probably have a fairly high tolerance to pain as well. As long as you have no adverse side effects to CBD, and you're not on other prescribed medications, jump to a higher dosage. If you're consuming it once a day and you want to be conservative, try adding an additional 5mg each serving and keep track of what is happening on your battlefield. Your body will tell you.

If All Else Fails:

Experiment with different or maybe multiple delivery systems. Sprays, edibles & topicals may work just as well as suppositories and vapes. One size does not fit all!

There is a sixth possible reason. It is not the topic of this book, but at some point (usually years in the future,) the effectiveness of CBD may feel like it has lost some of its strength. Well, the truth is, CBD is most effective when it has a small amount of THC combined with it. The two together have a synergistic effect that is very powerful on the body and the endocannabinoid system.

If you are unable to find relief, the next step is to reach out to a doctor or nurse who has the medical experience of using Cannabis/Hemp CBD who can spend one-on-one time with you and work closely with you to find the right solution to your pain-needs.

If you need help finding a physician or medical practitioner that prescribes Cannabis/Hemp Cannabinoids for pain management, check my website or contact me directly, and I'll send you some recommendations.

Email: inforequest@thecbdwriter.com
Website: https://thecbdwriter.com

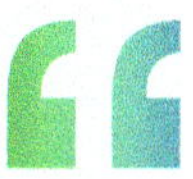

ACUTE PAIN SUFFERERS

AFTER A TRAUMA, USE CBD LONG ENOUGH FOR THE BODY TO HEAL ITSELF FROM THE INJURY. ONCE THE BODY HAS RECOVERED, DECREASE YOUR INTAKE OVER A TWO OR THREE DAY PERIOD, THEN STORE THE UNUSED CBD CONTENTS IN A COOL DARK PLACE AND USE AS NEEDED, IF NEEDED. DISCARD OIL AFTER 12 MONTHS.

CHAPTER TWO

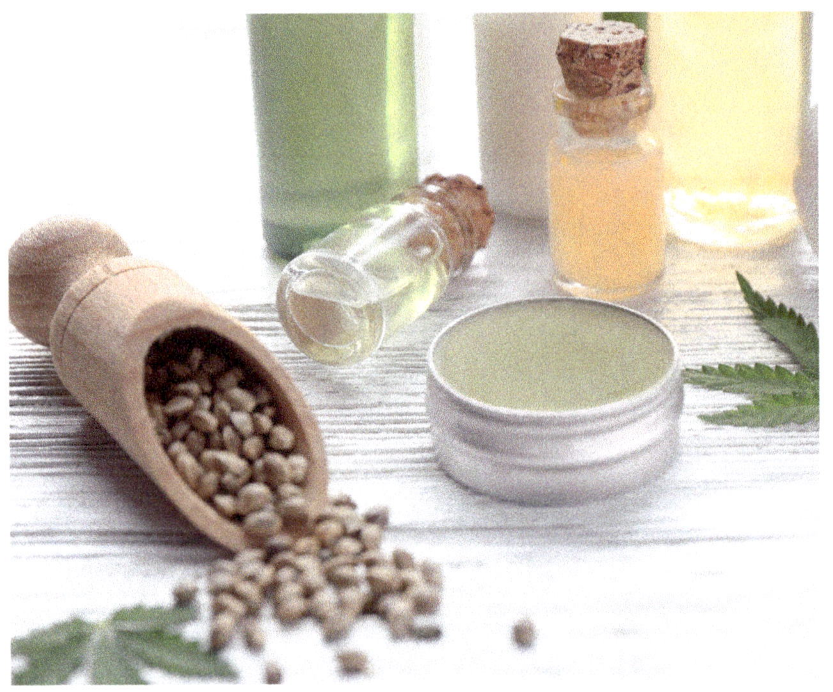

How to use CBD?

Methods For Absorbing CBD And Managing Pain

DOSAGE

Whether you're experienced or a first-time user, understanding the complexity of how CBD works and the various methods of application can be extremely confusing, especially since the industry is so new.

When it comes to how much CBD to use, start slow and increase gradually.

While there are 100's of articles about the benefits and results of CBD, there are few about properly dosing CBD.

The Food and Drug Administration (FDA) has been authorized by Congress to create and standardize "Recommended Daily Intakes." (RDI) This defines the "daily levels" of nutrients that are sufficient enough to meet the requirements of 97%-98% of healthy individuals in the United States.

To make things more confusing, unlike with other supplements, the FDA has not created an RDI for CBD, which means CBD does not have an "official" serving size.

There are a large number of factors affecting the size of the dosage amount that will work for you. The quality and potency of the CBD intake will undoubtedly influence what you feel, but other factors to consider include:

- Your weight
- Your metabolism
- Your diet
- The condition being treated
- The severity of your illness
- Your tolerance to CBD

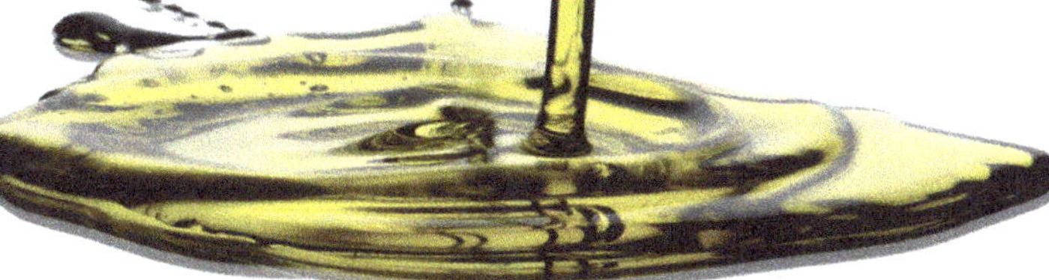

How to Choose Your CBD Dosage

So how much CBD should you take then? Here are a couple of easy tips to get you started.

"Cannabinoid medicine is still in its infancy; thus, dosing is not necessarily scientifically based, and confusion is common among healthcare providers. However, unlike marijuana and THC, the risks associated with CBD are extremely low, with not a single case report of CBD overdose in the literature. Regardless, the dose of CBD should be titrated to effect, emphasizing the adage "START LOW, GO SLOW." - Michael E. Schatman, PhD

Body Weight

Pain Severity	<25lbs	26-45lbs	46-85lbs	85-150lbs	151-240lbs	>241lbs
Moderate	1.5 mg	6 mg	9 mg	12 mg	18 mg	22.5 mg
Severe	6 mg	9 mg	12 mg	15 mg	22.5 mg	30 mg
Chronic	9 mg	12 mg	15 mg	18 mg	27 mg	45 mg

Pain Management CBD Dosage Body Weight Calculater

1. Estimate your dosage based on your body weight

As with all prescribed medications, a person with more body weight will need to have more mg's of CBD to experience its effects. A general rule of thumb for determining your personal CBD serving size is to start by taking 1–6mgs of CBD for every 10 pounds of body weight you have based on your level of pain.

For example, 20mg-33mg might be a good starting dose for a 200lb patient, while 15mg-25mg would have a similar effect on a person who weighs 150lb.

If you're determining your initial dosage based on your weight, gauge how your body reacts to the amount of mg's of CBD taken. If your pain decreases say 50% then increase another 2-5mg's and monitor your body's reaction.

2. Estimate your dosage based on milligrams

A second method would be to start out with 5-10mg, gauge your body's reaction, stay at that level for at least a week for your body to get used to ingesting a new supplement and then increase from there.

Once you find your personal serving size, you can adjust the dosage on days where pain gets out of control. There is no one ideal CBD serving, and with time, you will learn how your body reacts to a CBD supplement.

Keeping Track

Doctors are successful at treating patients because they keep a written history of each visit. When treating a person's physical ailments doctors will use a "Take 2 Aspirin and call me in the morning approach," meaning based on the results of the amount of aspirin taken the night or the period of time before, the doctor will prescribe a higher or lower dosage to get his desired effect in his patient.

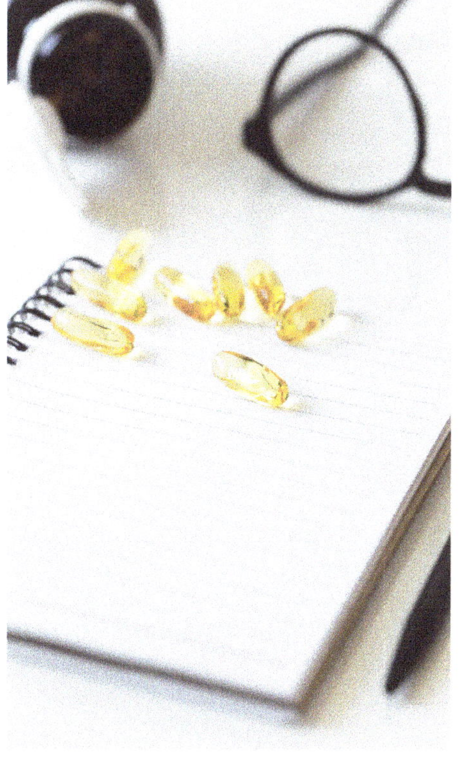

New discoveries in medicine and the human body are exciting, and the discovery of the endo-cannabinoid system and how it interacts with our bodies haven't even scratched the surface yet.

Grab yourself a fresh new notepad and pay attention to what is going on in your body. Get yourself some self-stickie tabs that you can use to create sections. Each section will be based on your personal needs, so no two personal histories will be the same.

"There is a growing body of evidence to suggest that cannabinoids are beneficial for a range of clinical conditions, including pain & inflammation."

- Cannabinoid Delivery Systems for Pain and Inflammation Treatment. MDPI

Here is how you might break down what is going on in your body.

Section 1: Symptoms

- What's causing them
- How long have I had the problem
- What have I tried
- Other pertinent notes
- Do vitamins help
- Do I have prescriptions
- What are the side effects

Section 2: CBD Consumption

- Starting day 1
- Starting dosage amount
- How much taken, how many mg's
- What taken
- Did I feel anything
- Did I start out with too much
- Did I experience any side effects
- Am I finding any relief

Section 3: Goals

- I want to walk two miles
- I want to roller blade
- I want to bowl
- If I could only...
- And so on and so on

You will create sections for your history based on what's important to you. Each of us have a different hurdle to climb over, some have high mountainous regions while others have little hiccups.

Important, Importante, Adviso

Date everything, and maybe if it's important enough to you timestamp it as well. Why not, it will become something very significant in your future when it comes to all the data you've gathered over the years.

Keep notes on for example, if you start with 25mg, what do you feel throughout the first few minutes after taking, and then the rest of the day. Do you notice little changes occurring either immediately or over time, do you feel uplifted and alert after taking, do you feel drowsy, do you feel immediate relief from pain or do you sense a gradual relief over a period of time?

These are all important notes to put into your personal history. CBD aids in reducing inflammation. So if you don't feel immediate relief, work at it. Explore what works for you. Start slow and grow from there.

TAKING CBD
THROUGH
ORAL ADMINISTRATION

Oral definition from Wikipedia: "Oral administration" is a route of administration where a substance is taken through the mouth. Many medications are taken orally because they are intended to have a systemic effect, reaching different parts of the body via the bloodstream.

This is the unofficial pharmaceutical companies' product & profit development list/guide.

Enteral medications (defined as: medicine passing through the mouth naturally or artificially) come in various forms, including:

- Tablets to swallow, chew or dissolve in water or under the tongue
- Capsules and chewable capsules (with a coating that dissolves in the stomach or bowel to release the medication there)
- Time-release or sustained-release tablets and capsules (which release the medication gradually)
- Powders or granules
- Teas
- Drops
- Liquid medications or syrups

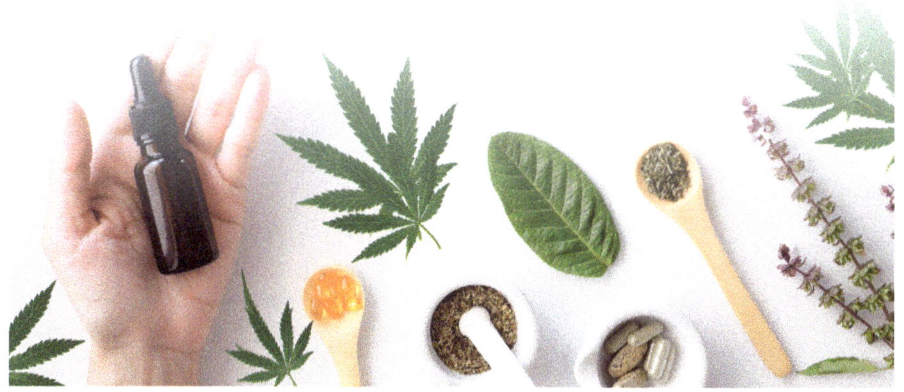

Why Is This Important To Humans

This list gives you and me the layman a categorized tree of medically possible ways for the human body to absorb CBD using oral administration. The onus is on getting the benefits of the plant into your bloodstream so you can get the pain relief you are seeking.

In a combined family of 12, I (David) am the only tea drinker. That works for me, but maybe not for you. Jessica, on the other hand, loves, and I emphasize, loves coffee and chocolate. Maybe capsules or drops work better for you. No one person is the same. This list gives us multiple ways to explore what works for each one of us individually, at our own pace.

Let's look at the 5 most common methods for taking CBD through oral administration.

This list is not in any particular order, and it is not extensive. They are fairly common enough that there isn't a need to put them in order.

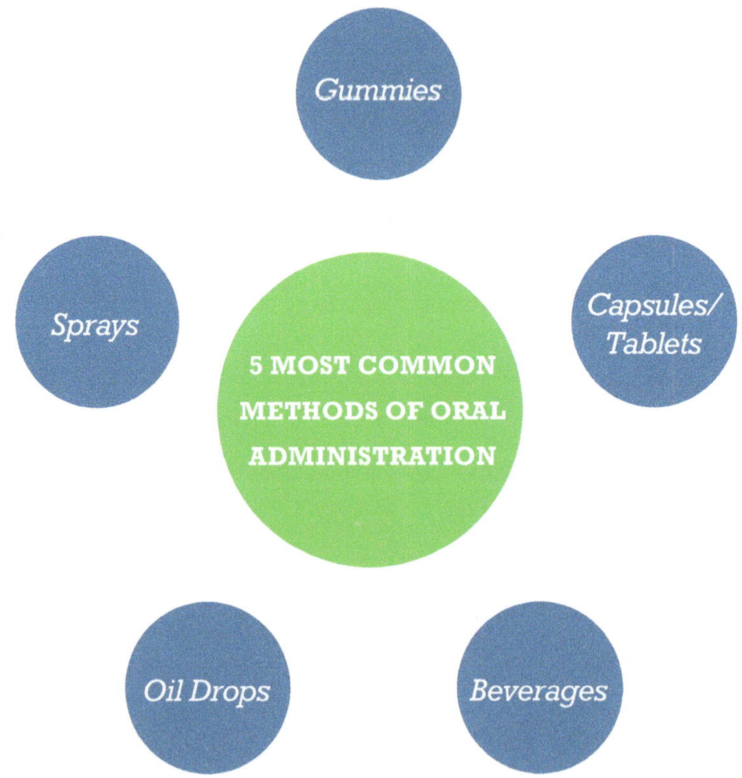

Gummies

If you liked to eat gummy bears as a kid, then you're going to love CBD gummies. They're a perfect combination of chewy texture and tangy fruit sweetness. Generally, they don't have a hemp aftertaste, just pure gummy flavor. They're the ideal choice for people who don't like the taste of CBD or hemp.

CBD Gummies are becoming very popular because they are convenient, discreet, fun, and a flavorful way to get your medicine. CBD Gummies can be made from hemp-based CBD or cannabis-based CBD. Only gummies without THC can be sold online.

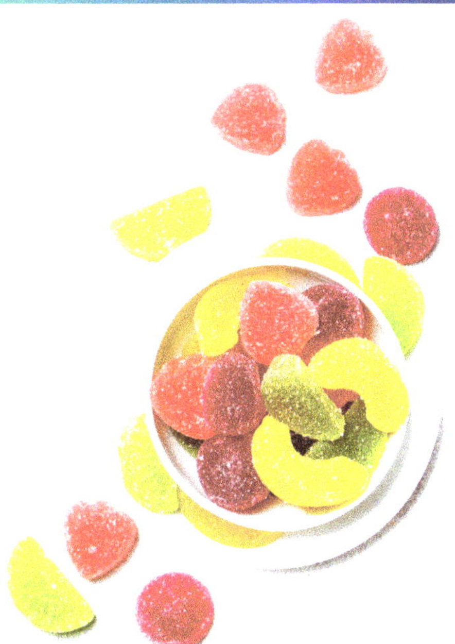

Taking CBD for pain can be as simple as snacking on a few tasty Gummies once or twice per day.

Similar to taking chewable vitamins, Gummies offer a safe, effective way for quickly consuming CBD as a daily supplement. You can find them available in a range of potencies from 5mg-25mg and are typically sold in 30-60 count resealable bags/bottles.

What To Look For In CBD Gummies

What to look for when evaluating your gummy is first the quality of the cannabidiol.

Where did they come from, are there any third party lab tests you can reference?

Lastly, how much CBD do you want in each gummy or each serving?

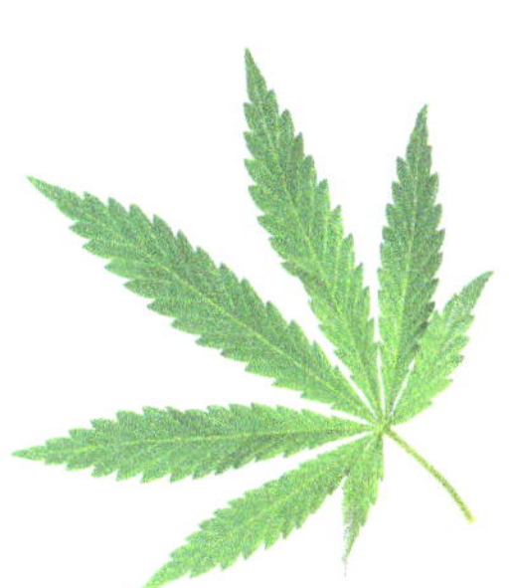

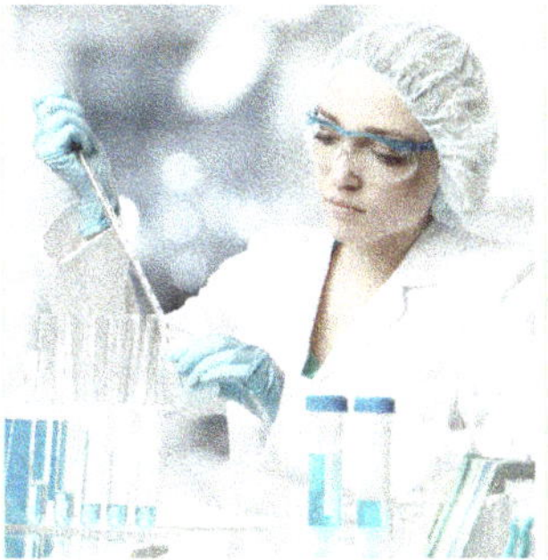

Servings per container 15

Serving Size 2 Pieces (4.5g)

Amount per serving

Calories 15

% Daily Value*

Total Fat 0g	0%
Saturated Fat 0g	0%
Trans Fat 0g	
Cholesterol 0mg	0%
Sodium 15mg	1%
Total Carbohydrate 3 g	1%
Dietary Fiber 0g	0%
Total Sugars 2g	
Inclues 2g Added Sugars	4%
Protein 0g	

Vitamin D 0mcg 0%	•	Calcium 0mg 0%
Iron 0mg 0%	•	Potassium 0mg 0%
Vitamin C 10mg 10%		

Capsules/Tablets

CBD capsules, soft gels, and tablets can be a convenient way to take this popular form of the supplement. There's no hemp aftertaste, and you avoid the sugar found in edibles like CBD gummies. Taking a capsule can be very discreet as well since most of these capsules simply look like any other over-the-counter supplement or vitamin.

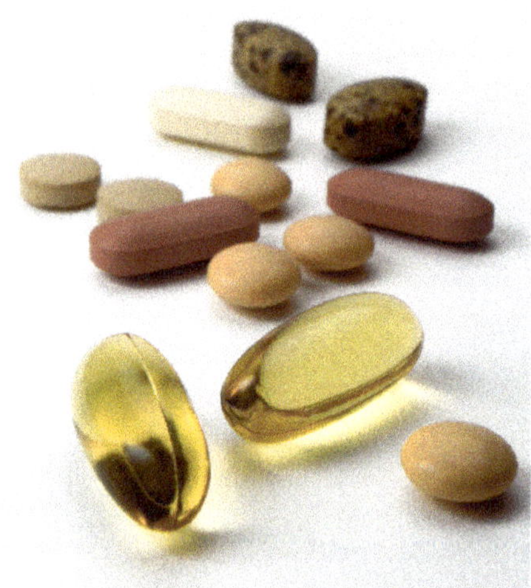

WORD OF CAUTION:
Something to remember when starting with CBD.

Each person's body reacts differently to cannabidiol, and it is possible for people to have side effects, as mentioned earlier. It's also common for people to respond differently to taking CBD in different forms, so you might feel differently after taking capsules versus swallowing CBD oil or vaping CBD. You may want to start with a lower dosage when trying a new way of ingesting CBD for the first time.

Beverages

CBD drinks are nothing more than drinks that contain CBD. As with other forms mentioned in this book, people are drinking CBD to provide themselves with relief from some type of health ailment, such as our focus - pain.

CBD drinks are probably the easiest of all to get a healthy dose of CBD into your system. Drinks are an excellent source for people who do not enjoy the taste of CBD oil.

Check out the available varieties on the next page.

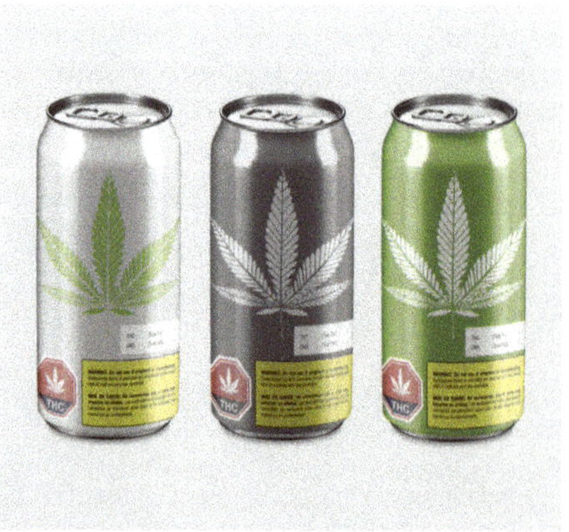

Note: The Entourage Effect, CBD Drinks & Other Intake Methods

In 2015 researchers analyzing and studying the medicinal properties of the cannabis plant at the Hebrew University of Jerusalem's Lautenberg Center for General and Tumor Immunology discovered what is known today as the "entourage effect."

In laymen terms, the entourage effect is where many cannabinoids, flavonoids, terpenes, work together synergistically to formulate a stronger encounter with the human body and its receptors as opposed to just using CBD as a single component.

This entourage effect gained a lot of attention in the medical cannabis community, and many of the CBD beverage companies with CBD product manufacturers are using the entourage effect to maximize the effectiveness of their product; thus they infuse their drinks and products with several elements, not just CBD by itself.

"I don't think we have that many good drugs for pain, and we know that CBD has fewer side effects than Opioids"

\- Daniel Clauw, MD

CBD Drink Manufacturers Are Creating Some Pretty Amazing Drinks.

Existing beverages available today:

- Water
- Flavored Water
- Carbonated Flavored Waters
- CBD-Infused Sodas
- CBD Energy Drinks
- Hemp Beers/IPA's
- CBD Coffees
- Sparkling Tonics
- CBD Teas

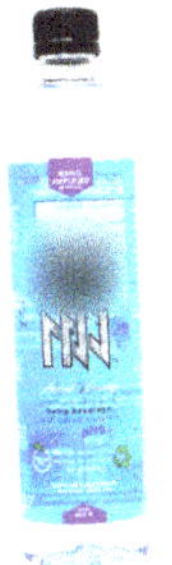
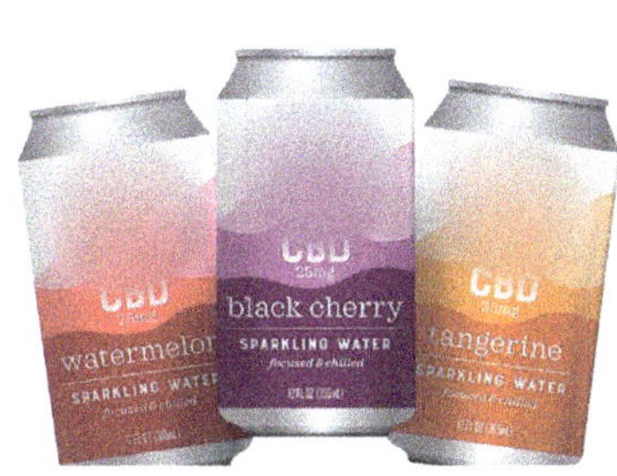

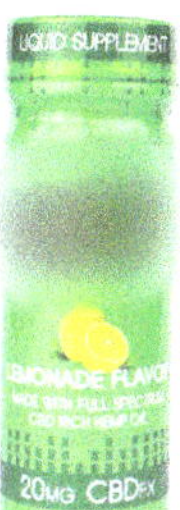

Please do not purchase these samples, they have not been properly vetted to make sure they meet all of the standards that I'm talking about in this book. These are for illustrative purposes only.

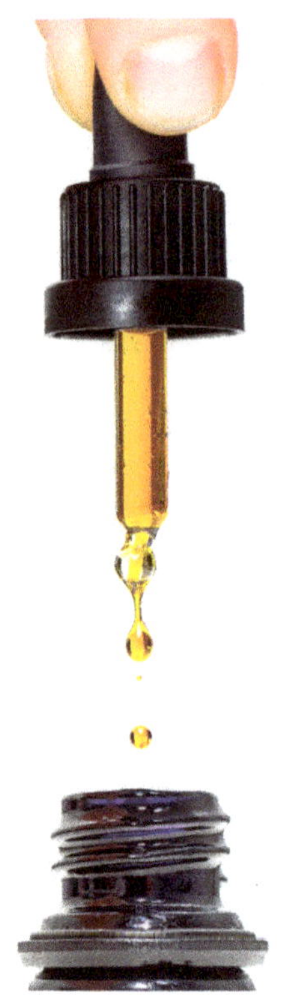

HOW TO USE CBD

Oil Drops

A person can use CBD oil in a multitude of ways to find relief from various symptoms, but first, it needs to be harvested and extracted. The oil is extracted from the hemp plant, but it can be manufactured synthetically as well. I don't know if synthetic is any good, but me, I'll stick with the real plant.

Harvesting CBD oil is a process where they use extraction solvents to separate and collect CBD oils from the seeds and the stalks. Testing the extracted oil for CBD (cannabidiol content) is the next step in the process, this is how they know the content and quality of the extract. The oil goes through additional steps of processing before it is used. See endnotes page for additional information.

At the moment, oil has become the preferred mode of administration for many medicinal users because that mode has been around the longest, and is most well known.

FYI, concentrated extracts allow for the consumption of larger doses of cannabinoids in easily ingestible forms. With CBD oil, there is no risk of intoxication (getting high), so more substantial doses of it can be consumed. (Note: within the parameters of what works for you.)

Some people prefer a holistic approach to health and may worry about the stigma associated with using "Pot." Well CBD is not Pot, and CBD oil has no odor that would smell or identify a consumer as a cannabis user. You can use it discretely in pretty much any social setting.

The beautiful thing about oil's or tinctures is it is easy to measure the amount you want to consume regularly by counting "drops" or measuring "volume."

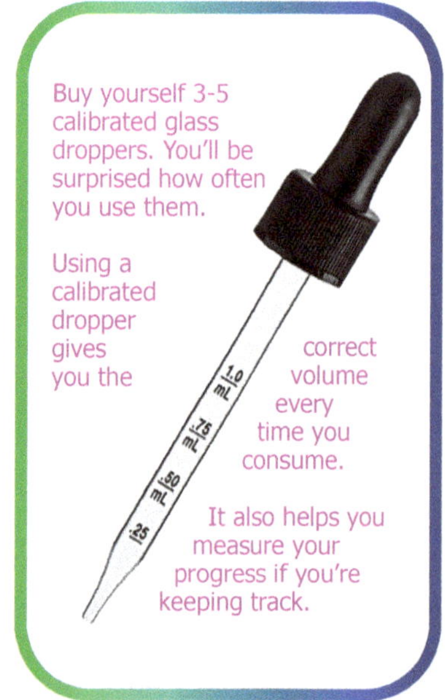

Oral Sprays

Sprays can deliver a high-level dose of CBD into your mouth each time you spray, allowing for a very effective method of absorption. What can be challenging with tinctures, drops, and sprays are determining how much CBD you are actually consuming, from either the dropper or each spray, because most bottles out there only show the total CBD content and don't list the per-dose amount. That is not good!

Good manufacturers will list the amount of mg's in the bottle and how many mg's are delivered per spray or per use. Use the weight calculator on page 17 to calculate how much CBD

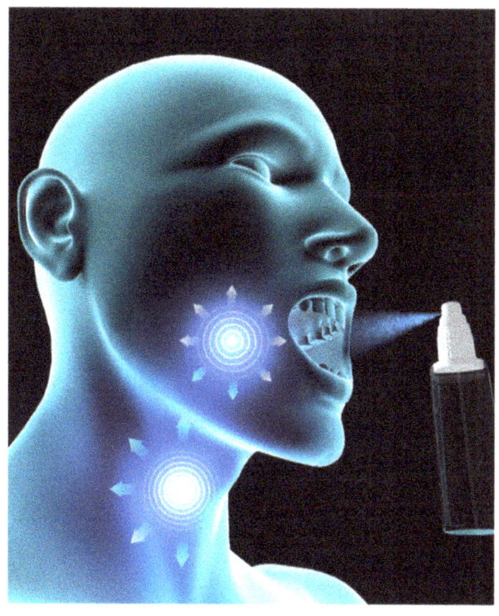

per dose to use. In regards to pricing, remember that the price per bottle could be more for a product that has a higher CBD content per dose.

Sprays also come in a variety of flavors, making it even more desirable to consume. Each manufacturer will design and create CBD sprays with various ingredients to enhance the effectiveness of the spray. The spray's convenient means of ingestion also make it ideal for using it alongside other CBD products for even more significant benefits.

Using the spray is quite simple. Aim the nozzle into your mouth and spray your tongue with the number of sprays required to get the desired mg's of CBD. That's it.

Product Samples

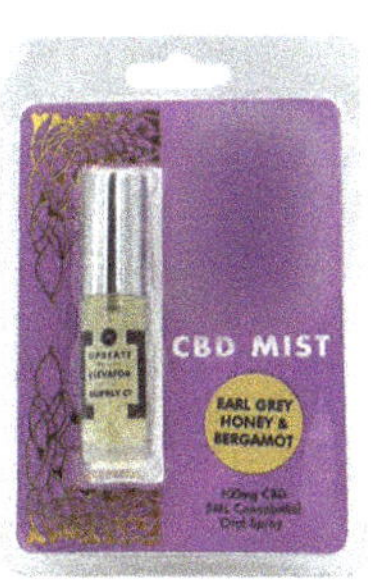
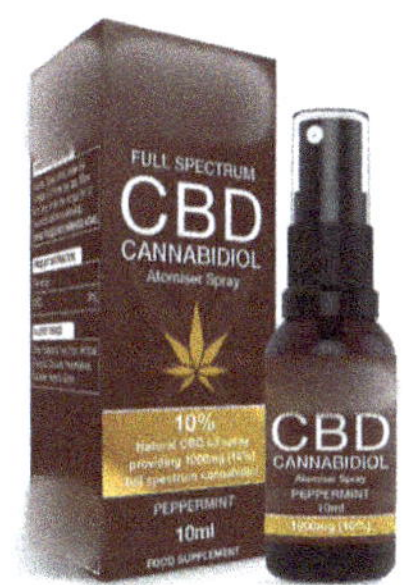
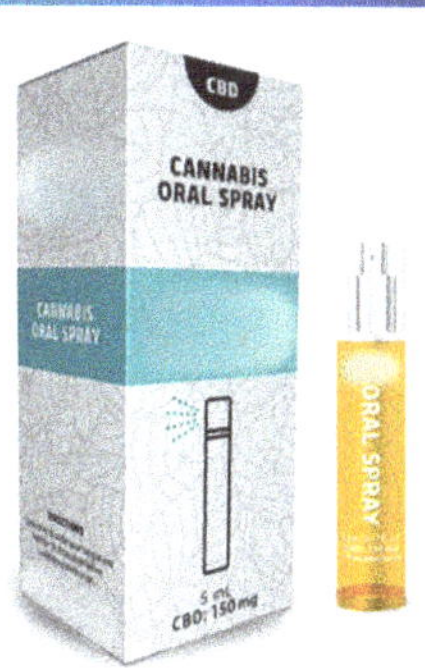

Please do not purchase these samples, they have not been properly vetted to make sure they meet all of the standards that I'm talking about in this book. These are for illustrative purposes only.

SUBLINGUAL OPTIONS

What is a sublingual?

We'll use Wikipedia again. Here is the accepted general definition of what a sublingual is.

Sublingual (abbreviated SL), from the Latin for "under the tongue", refers to the pharmacological route of administration by which substances diffuse into the blood through tissues under the tongue.

Two ways to utilize your mouth for intake of CBD.

Consuming through the mouth into the digestive system, CBD will slowly work its way into your bloodstream, and eventually, the effects will be felt. Conversely, when CBD oil is administered sublingually, it's held under your tongue for anywhere from 30 to approximately 90 seconds so that the capillaries and the mucous membranes under your tongue can absorb the oil's active ingredients.

The benefit of consuming CBD sublingually is that the absorption process bypasses the digestion and the liver, allowing the CBD to reach your bloodstream and interact with your endocannabinoid system much more quickly.

For those looking for quick effects, a sublingual CBD oil or product is ideal.

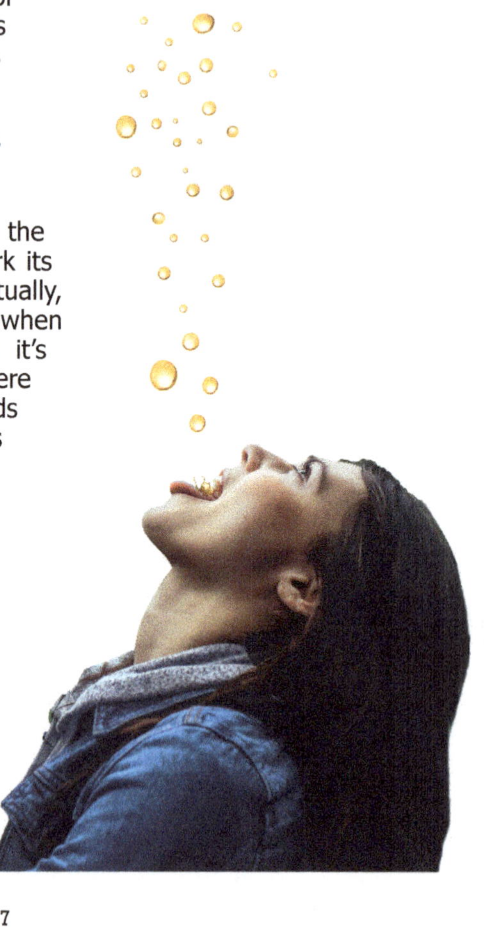

EDIBLES

A popular method for taking CBD is consuming edible products made with CBD Concentrate. CBD edibles are basically "any food item" that is specifically CBD-infused. Don't run to a dispensary and grab the first edible you can find. You should know the basics of how CBD edibles work first.

Also, make sure you purchase an edible product that's high in quality and potent enough to do what it claims. Remember, read your labels before purchasing.

Ingesting CBD takes a little longer for the effects to be felt, because medications as well as CBD that is ingested, must pass through the digestive system and the liver before the cannabinoids reach the receptors, the brain, and the areas of inflammation.

CBD vapes and tinctures can take effect within minutes because of how quickly it enters the bloodstream. CBD edibles, on the other hand, can take anywhere from thirty minutes to two hours to take effect. How long it takes for edibles to be felt depends on the state of your digestive system and other factors as pointed out on page 16.

The effects of CBD edibles are not as noticeable as those of THC edibles. You will not "trip out" or feel high in the traditional sense of the phrase.

Remember, the point of taking CBD edibles is not to alter your state of mind or mood, but to remove your body's distractions to bring healing, to bring you to a place of less or no pain.

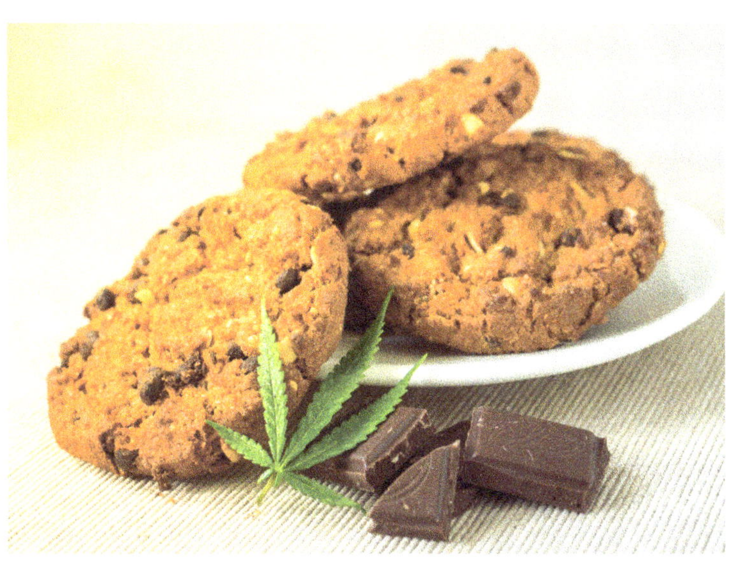

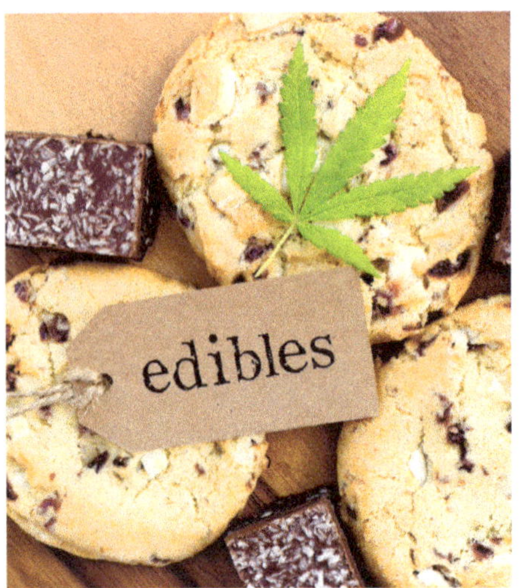

CBD edibles may take a more extended amount of time to be felt, but the benefits of ingesting CBD allows for the effects to come on a little more slowly.

The most important thing I think is that its effects last longer. Because of this long-lasting effect, CBD edibles and the slow release of CBD may be a great way to keep your pain at bay for longer. Plus, by micro-dosing your edibles, you can make sure the CBD is released regularly throughout the day.

Micro-dosing means eating a small amount at regular intervals during your day.

When starting something new like CBD edibles, remember to start with a small dosage and work up to a place that is comfortable for you.

Document the what, how much, and when you've taken your edible(s).

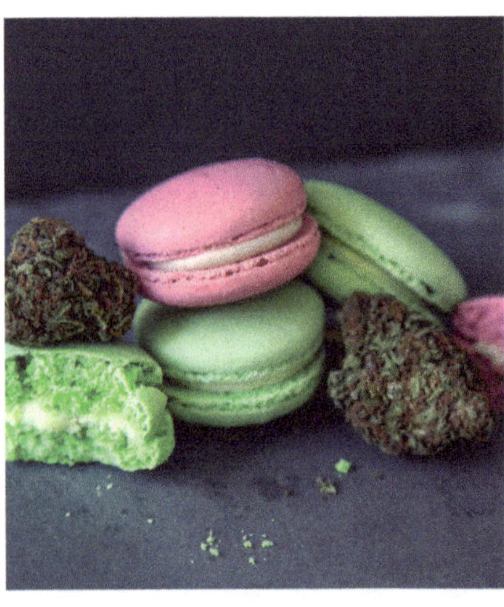

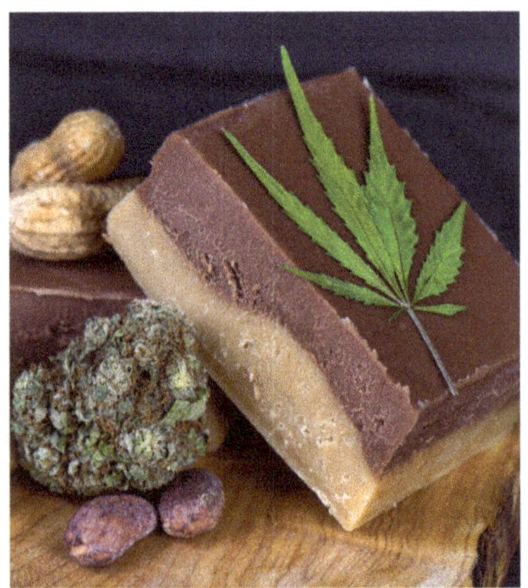

INHALING

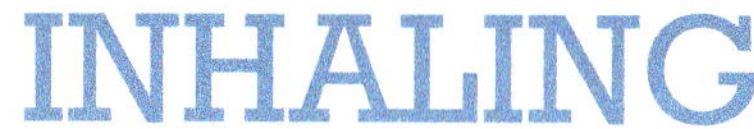

There are basically two methods to consume CBD when it comes to inhaling. There are others, but those are for another book on more advanced topics. For this book, we'll focus on smoking the physical plant itself and using Vapes. I'll explain both types of ingestion, but they are still basically the same, inhaling.

Understand if you are not a smoker, I don't necessarily recommend that you take up smoking CBD cigarettes. But I do agree that vaping might be an excellent alternative to smoking the plant. Both take an adjustment to use and getting used to. Smoking is an acquired taste and not meant for everybody.

Now on the flip side, if you are a smoker or ex-smoker and don't mind smoking pre-rolled CBD joints, then you might have an excellent way to get the plants benefits into you quickly.

Once you get past the "first time smoking" or "coughing" then consuming CBD via smoking really isn't a big deal.

Again smoking is an acquired taste or activity, but generally a good way to consume hemp plant CBD.

HOW TO USE CBD

How to Inhale CBD

If you're a new smoker or considering becoming a new smoker, here are some of the various options available to you:

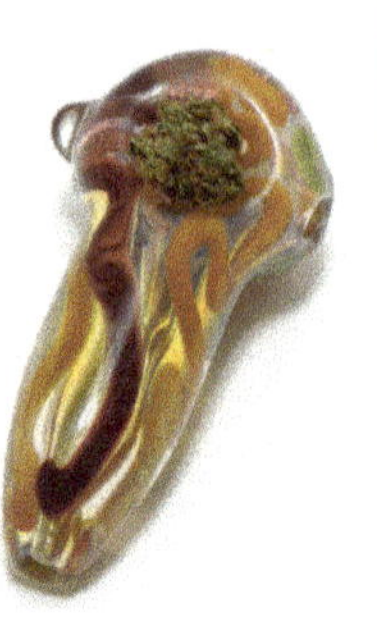

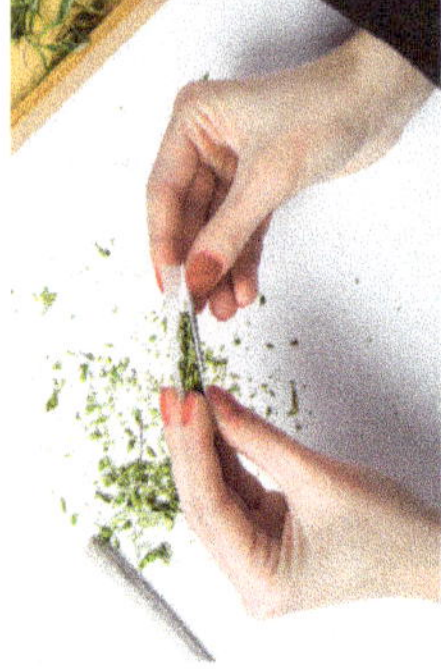

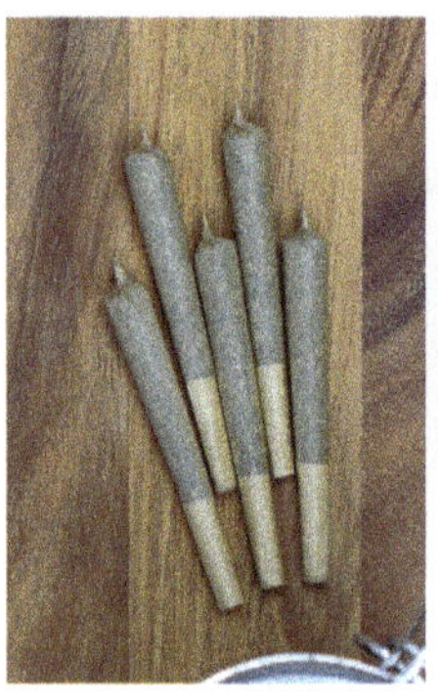

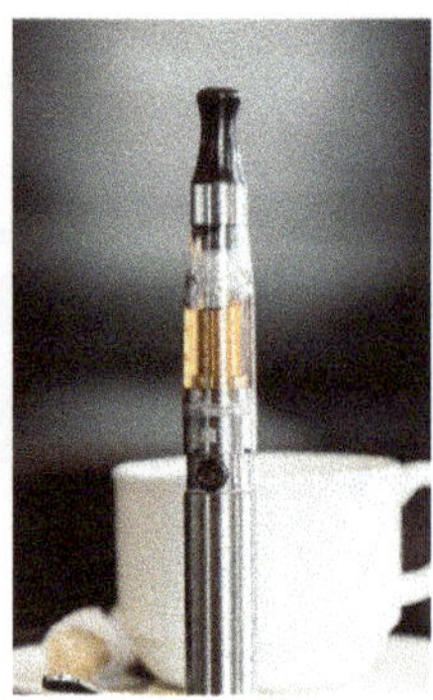

A Pipe or Water Pipe to smoke

Rolling Papers (Rolling it yourself)

Pre-Roll Joints Ready to Smoke

A Vape Cartridge With Battery

What's more, inhalation is one of the most convenient methods for people to get cannabis – in our case, CBD – into the body. Other than injection, inhalation is one of the faster delivery methods into the bloodstream.

The onset of the effects usually occurs within 5-10 minutes and can last for up to 2 hours

Smoking the Plant

Hemp, once it is harvested, is dried and prepared for medicinal use. If you purchase it in plant form, then you will put it in a pipe or roll it into a cigarette form and then smoke it. In cigarette form, mentally break it into quarters and start by smoking 1/4 at a time until you understand how it's impacting you. In a pipe, fill the bowl with a small amount and start with 3-6 puffs. This may feel odd to some of you, but remember you are not smoking to get high, you're smoking for relief.

Keep your history when you smoke. Write down everything. You'll learn a lot about yourself.

VAPING

Vaping is another popular method for CBD intake, but to a new consumer, I'm sure it will raise many questions. I understand that out of all means available to consume CBD, vaping is the most unfamiliar to new consumers. However, vaping presents unique benefits that both new and experienced CBD consumers should consider.

When you vaporize the terpenes and cannabinoids, as we mentioned on page 24, the consumer receives all the entourage effects of the residual cannabinoids, terpenes, and other compounds gassing off without the harshness of inhaling ignited smoke from the plant.

Vaping allows for the effects of the medication to be felt quickly, without the adverse effects that can come with smoking. Vaping is particularly helpful when you need fast-acting relief from pain and inflammation.

A Note About Inhaling Vapes

The vape battery heats either a single or dual coil, the oil drops onto the coil, combusts, causing a vapor that can be inhaled. Beginners can inhale too much at one time in the beginning and may experience harsh stinging sensations that can irritate the throat and lungs. Start slow. Experienced users the same goes for you. A large intake can make you cough and choke, so take your time to get the feel of how vaping works and makes you feel.

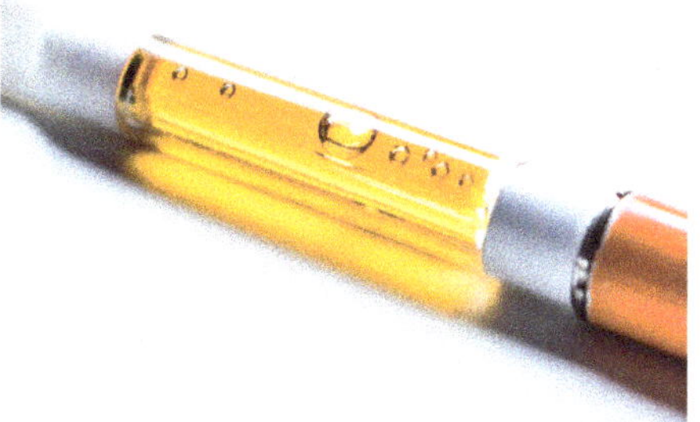

Cartridge ready to vape immediately

When smoking or vaping your CBD cart, make sure you follow the dosing instructions given or figure out how many mg's you need. If you pick a product without dosing instructions, then use the dosing instructions at the beginning of this chapter and then consume as desired.

When purchasing vapes, you can buy them in cartridge form, or you can buy refillable cartridges and purchase the oil and refill as needed.

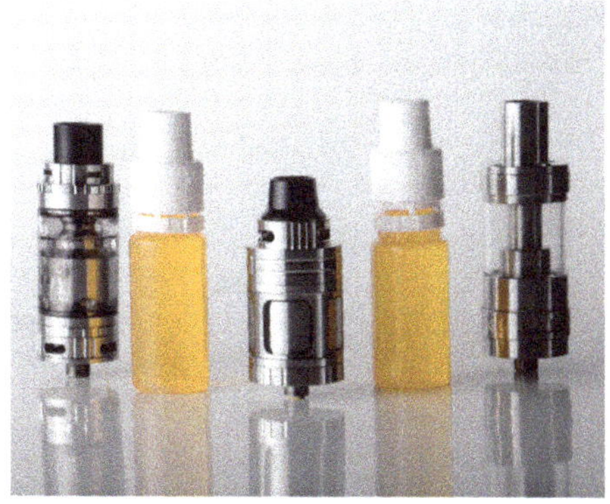

Refillable cartridge for oil

7 Ways to Manage Pain with CBD

TOPICALS
AND WHAT
ARE
THEY?

When it comes to pain relief, like aching muscles or muscle spasms, arthritis, joint pain, back pain, etc., when you put some form of ointment such as Bengay or Biofreeze on the affected area(s), this is called a topical. When putting on hand lotion for your dry hands, this is a topical.

CBD INFUSED TOPICALS

Today we have what we call "topicals infused with CBD." These topicals are Cannabidiol (CBD)-infused lotions, and oils that are absorbed through the skin for local relief of pain, soreness, and inflammation.

Because they're not psychoactive, (meaning you don't get high) patients can get the therapeutic benefits of the cannabis plant without the "high" or "euphoria" associated with other delivery methods such as inhaling and smoking by using CBD-infused topicals.

A word about strain-specific topicals. They attempt to harness or capture certain terpenes and cannabinoids in a specific chemical profile. (Because they affect the body and brain in different ways.) Then along with CBD and other cannabinoids, topical producers/manufacturers will then include other ingredients and essential oils for additional relief, such as cayenne pepper, wintergreen, and clove to create a new cannabis-infused product.

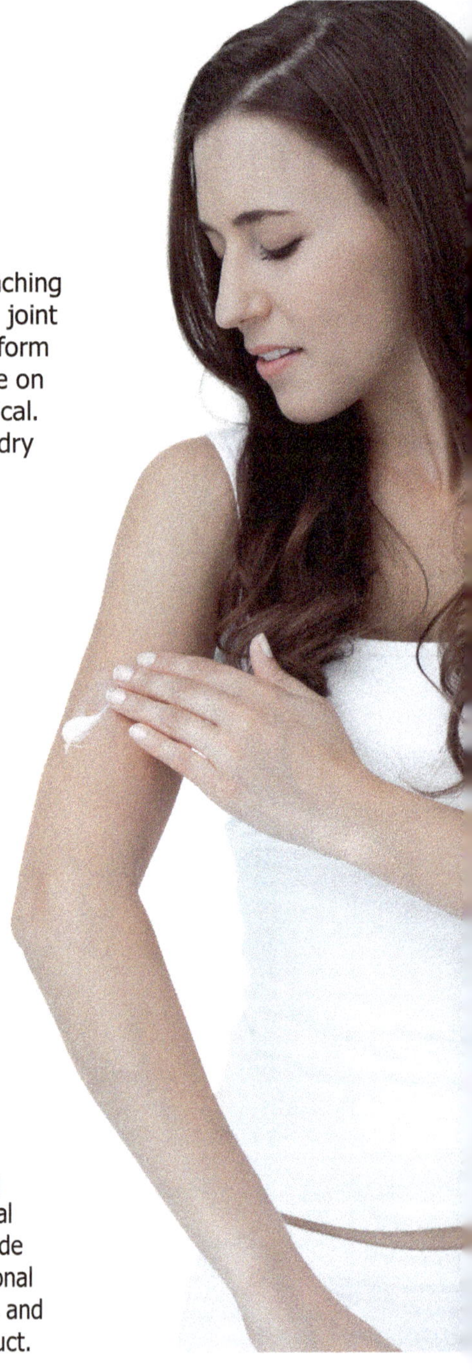

TYPES OF MEDICAL TOPICAL APPLICATIONS

- Topical solution
- Lotion
- Shake lotion
- Cream
- Ointment
- Gel
- Foam
- Transdermal patch
- Powder
- Solid
- Sponge
- Tape
- Vapor
- Paste
- Tincture

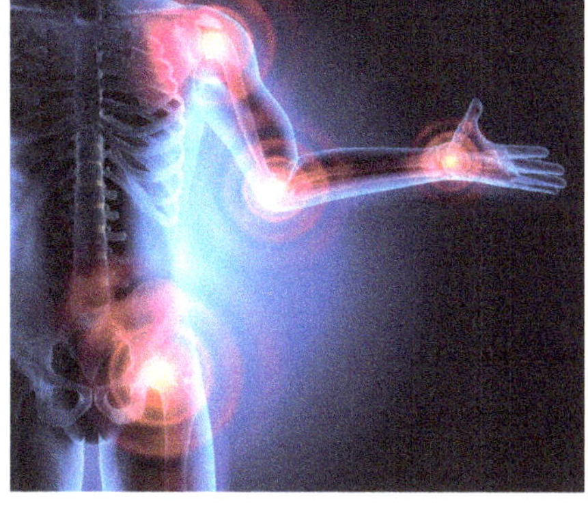

How Topicals Work

Your endocannabinoid system regulates your appetite, your mood, and your pain/pleasure receptors, among other things. These active cannabis plant compounds, THC and CBD, for example, are the chemicals that activate that system. These are the two prominent cannabinoids.

Keep this in the back of your mind. Your brain also manufactures its own version of cannabinoids including Anandamide which is similar to THC. THC/CBD and cannabinoids are all similar in that they all bind to your CB1 and CB2 receptors.

These receptors and the molecules that bind to them are responsible for a wide range of biological functions, such as anti-inflammation and pain relief.

"The most effective neuropathic pain relief occurs after 1 week of daily CBD treatment."

- Senior author Gabriella Gobbi, MD, PhD, professor of psychiatry, Neurobiological Psychiatry Unit, McGill University, Montreal Canada

When you use a CBD-infused topical product, CBD will bind directly to the receptors present in skin, muscle tissues, and nerves, and that brings relief to the inflamed area. It also makes its way into the bloodstream, where it interacts with CB2 receptors.

Topical CBD can and probably will get distributed to the rest of the body via the bloodstream if you use enough, but this happens so slowly that most people don't detect any mental effect.

Based on anecdotal reports, if the topical you're using is CBD with 0.3% THC or less, there will be no psychoactive side effects. Since there's usually no high, topicals are a great choice for people who want the relief without the intoxicating side effects, and personally speaking, I will feel relief from pain within minutes of using a good quality topical.

Why Use Topicals?

Short Answer, Relief From Pain and Inflammation Quickly

There is so much to learn about CBD. But we do know this, that it is a potent anti-inflammatory. When mixed with topical applications, it can directly treat pain, many times right at the source. Studies are beginning to show cannabis is much better for treating chronic pain, better than heavy narcotics.

Seniors, you know joint pain and arthritis are caused by inflammation. If you can target that inflammation with a topical, you should be able to find relief. A capsule of Oil in the Morning and a topical as needed could bring you much comfort.

Depending on the quality and potency, the effects of some Topicals can be felt right away, while others can take a little longer even up to a couple hours. Keep in mind that topicals will not get you high.

Word Of Caution: If you use a THC patch, you may feel some cerebral euphoria. Some transdermal patches allow THC to enter the bloodstream. Similarly, while many Topicals won't cause you to fail a drug test, there are no guarantees, so proceed accordingly.

Note: See the appendix for links to various case studies using CBD medicinally for pain.

Product Samples

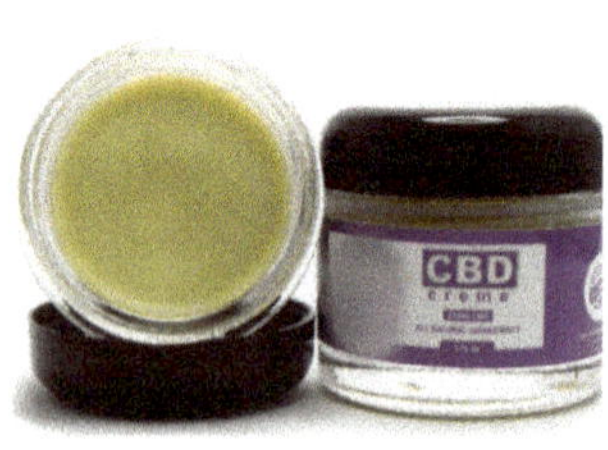
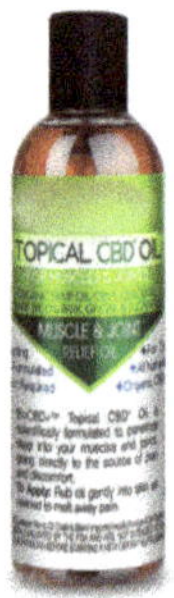
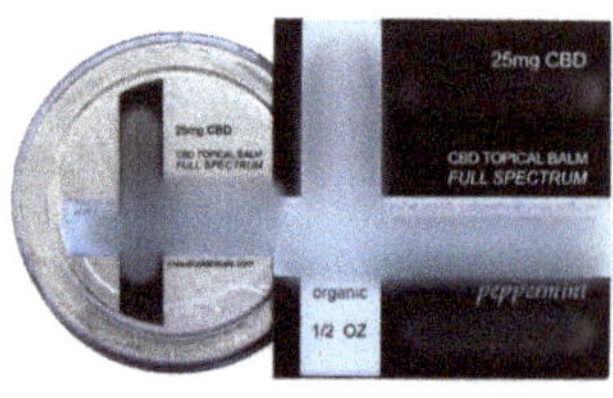

Please do not purchase these samples, they have not been properly vetted to make sure they meet all of the standards that I'm talking about in this book. These are for illustrative purposes only.

SUPPOSITORIES

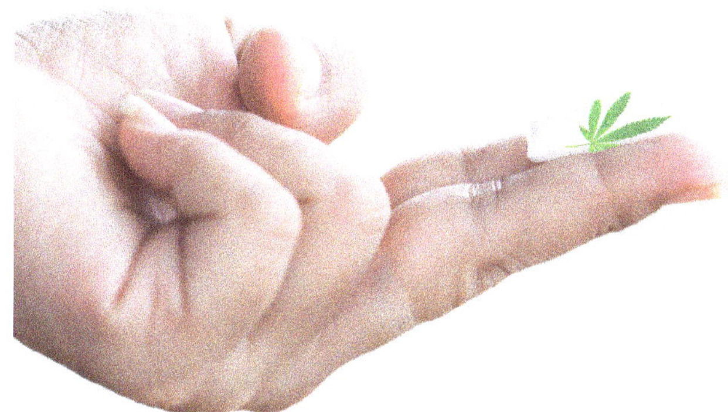

Okay, this is a topic that is generally considered taboo or frowned upon for open discussion in public circles. But generally, throughout history, suppositories have been one of the best methods to get medication into a person's bloodstream quickly via the rectum and/or vagina.

Suppositories, for the most part, look like miniature zeppelins. They're designed to be inserted into the rectum and then gradually melt by the heat of your body. The most common rectal CBD suppositories usually are about 2 grams and are roughly 2.5cm long.

Manufacturers will use cocoa butter, shea butter, coconut oil, or some combination mixed with CBD extract to deliver various dosage amounts almost immediately to your bloodstream. The impact should be felt rather quickly with the right dosage.

"Cannabis appears to be an effective pain management tool with few negative side effects." "The observed decrease in opiate usage among patients on cannabis therapy was the study's most striking finding. Again, 91 percent of survey respondents reported that they decreased the amount of opiates they were taking or eliminated them altogether."

- Cannabis In The Treatment Of Age-Related Pain
Survey Cannabis and Pain 2016

STEPS FOR SUPPOSITORY APPLICATION:

- First, always wash your hands in hot soapy water.

- If the suppository is room temperature or warmer place it in the back of the refrigerator for 15 minutes or under cold water until the suppository becomes firm.

- Carefully remove the suppository from the packaging. Don't break it or allow it to fall to the ground.

- If available you can use disposable gloves.

- Use a water-soluble lubricant and add a little to the tip of the suppository. Stay away from vaseline and petroleum-based lubricants. They will damage the medication.

- While lying on one side straighten out the bottom leg and pull your upper leg towards your chest area giving you easy access to expose the rectum.

- With the pointed end first, place suppository against your rectum and push with your finger until it passes through.

- Squeeze your buttocks together for a few moments and remain lying down for about 5 minutes to prevent the suppository from sliding out.

- Discard your used materials and wash your hands.

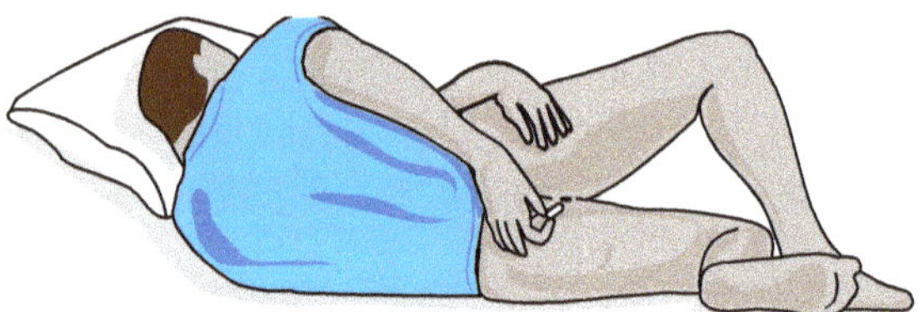

Dr. Paula-Noel Macfie PHD

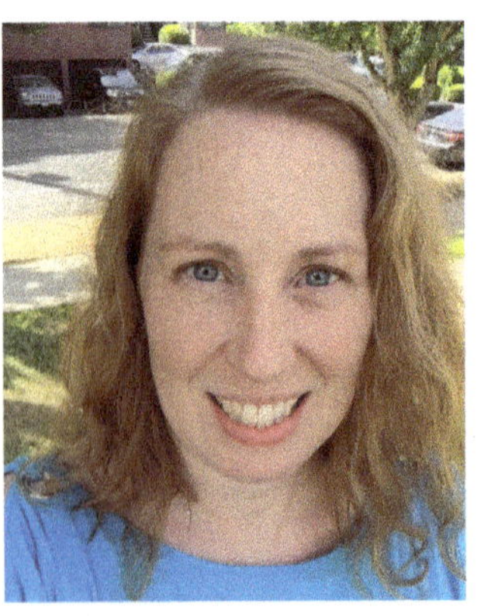

Her organization Back Door Medicine, is devoted to providing access to cannabis suppository information, education, and support

Dr. Paula-Noel Macfie explains the reason cannabis suppositories don't get you high:

"When administered rectally, the plant medicine directly enters the bloodstream through the cell walls and goes directly into the body, which is quickly distributed through the vascular system. It is a direct application to the bloodstream, bypassing the liver. The liver is a key to getting

high. THC travels through the liver to the brain to induce a head high. When smoked, it travels through the lungs to the villi, then on to the liver. When taking it orally, it makes its way to the liver through digestion. This method takes the longest because of the digestive process and the amount of travel it takes to get to the brain. In the brain, THC interacts with nerve receptors, causing euphoria. The bottom line: Cannabis suppositories allow for larger doses of plant medicine without the head high versus smoking and ingesting orally."

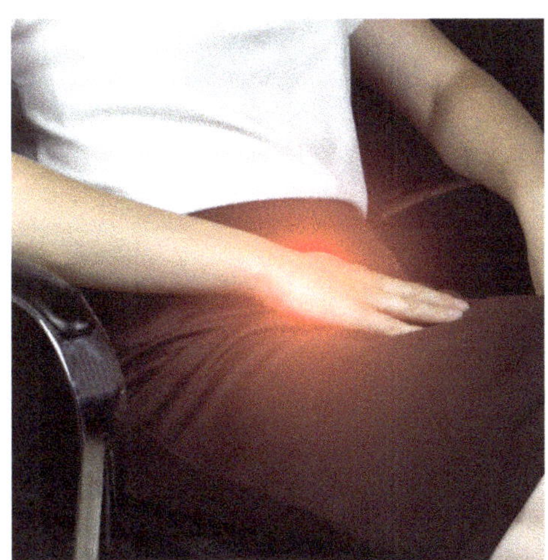

The super-fast absorption benefits of suppositories are gaining serious recognition in the medical marijuana community. This is an area that will see rapid growth as more high-quality products are brought to market in this form. Pain can be brought to a manageable place if not better with this method of use.

Though outside the focus of this book, ladies if you suffer from severe menstrual cramps or other female irregularities, look further into using a high-quality CBD suppository explicitly designed for the vagina.

Foria, a pretty well known manufacturer of sensual THC/CBD products explains:

"Within the female reproductive tract, endocannabinoid receptors are widespread. They are most dense in the uterus, but are also found in the fallopian tubes, ovaries, vagina and vulva. On a microscopic level, endocannabinoid receptors are located where they can exert control. They are associated with: (meaning to stimulate)

- nerves where they mediate sensations
- immune cells where they control inflammation
- glands where they influence hormone secretion
- muscles where they facilitate energy usage

There is only a sprinkling of research on this area, but ladies… use the information you learn here and apply it. If you can spend a little time exploring, you may find benefits that could change your life. But remember what Jessica derives from the use of the plant is different from what Sophia gets from the plant, which is different from what Brenda needs from the plant. Each person has different needs, so no two stories or histories are alike.

ISOLATES
AND
POWDERS

I do recognize powder isolates could and probably should come under the auspices of Oral Administration. But I put powder isolates as its own sub-topic because it can be used in so many different ways.

I'll summarize isolates like this. It can be used in almost every method we've discussed in this book. If you have the ability or would like the ability to mix and blend your own CBD healing creations for your individual pain relief or to sell as your own product, powder Isolate can fit that bill.

Isolates can be mixed into:

- drinks
- foods
- topicals
- balms
- smoothies
- tinctures
- and much more!

Powder isolates can be mixed with terpenes and other compounds to create a myriad of products.

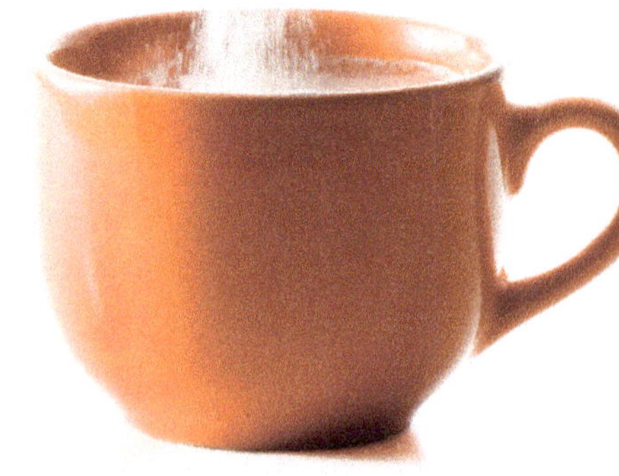

Isolate powder is a purified, crystallized form of CBD. It's a white powder striped of all other cannabinoids including the THC and other plant materials like terpenes, oils, and chlorophyll. What is left are naturally-derived CBD crystals that are odorless and flavorless. In this pure form, it's a very powerful anti-inflammatory.

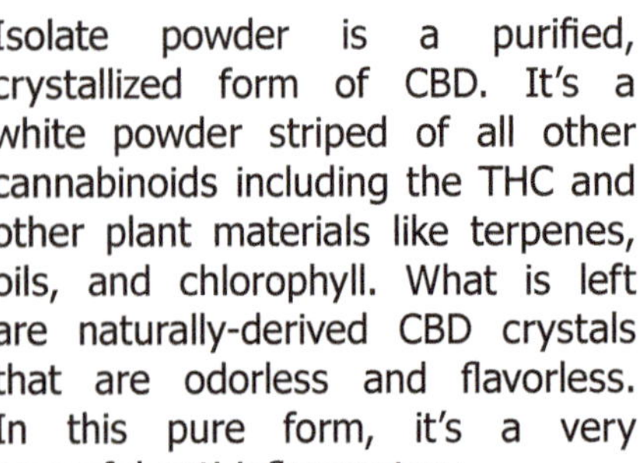

David Anthony Schroeder

CBD powder has many different uses for your daily routine, starting with edibles and drinks. But with a little knowledge and some experimentation, you can take your CBD consumption to a whole different level.

CBD is known for its long list of applications for providing relief and isolates have almost endless possible uses. You are only limited by what your mind can come up with.

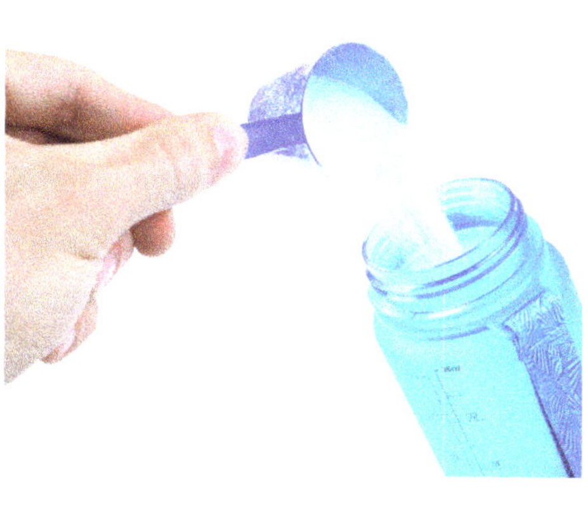

Some Possible Suggested Uses:

As a sub-lingual, try using a tiny measuring spoon like 1/32 of a teaspoon, or a stevia spoon, and grab a small amount of isolate or pinch enough Isolate between your fingers about the diameter of a AAA battery, pour or sprinkle it under your tongue and let it dissolve up to 90 seconds. Remember always to pay attention to the labels for recommended dosing instructions.

Since it's odorless and tasteless, there are many ways you can experiment with your daily dose(s). Try finding some recipes on the internet and cooking with it. Everybody enjoys some form of beverage, try working it into your favorite smoothie, coffee, or try creating something new. You may also sprinkle it over anything edible including yogurt and ice cream. Powder Isolate is very diverse, use it in everything daily.

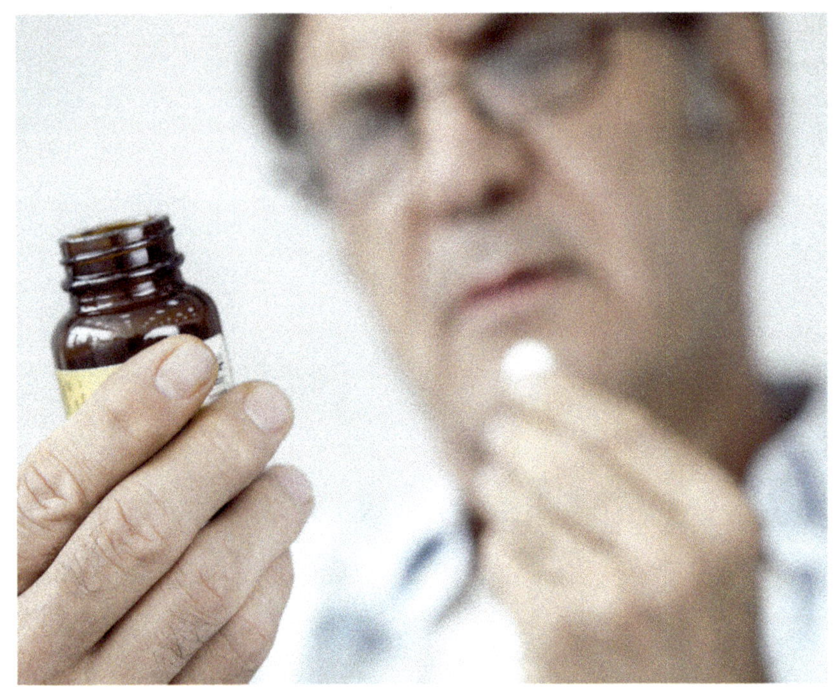

Reading Labels

READING LABELS

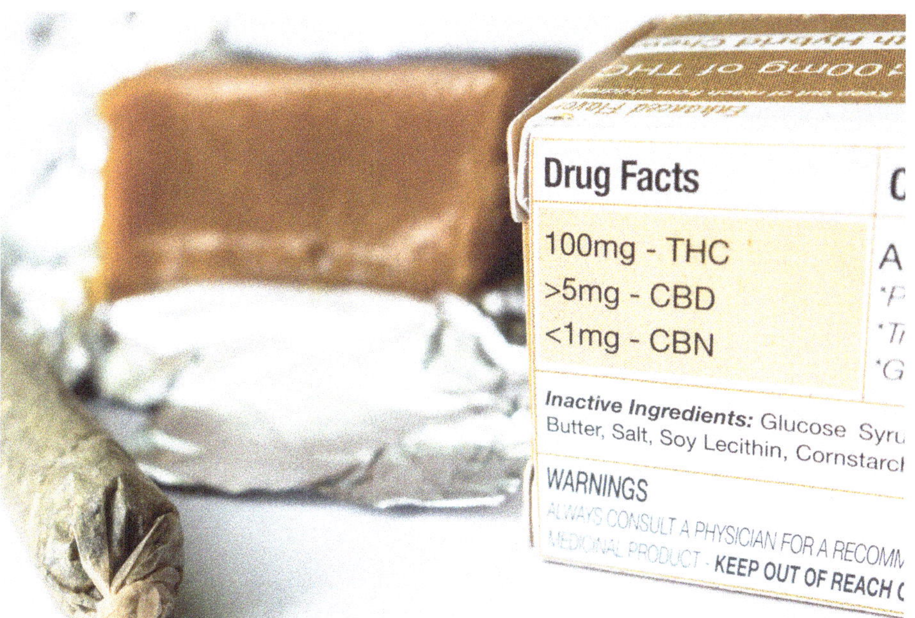

As of March 2020, the CBD industry is unregulated by the U.S. Food & Drug Administration (FDA), meaning they are completely hands off. The implications of no governmental oversite open's the door to "snake oil salesman" who sell a variety of "poor quality" CBD products. "Buyer, beware." As you begin this journey, you're going to see with your own eyes the lack of consistency across product labels.

CBD product labels will always feature the manufacturer and/or distributor of the CBD product. This allows you to dig in and research on your own to see whether a company is reliable and trustworthy. I recommend that you spend a little time looking into the company's testing standards.

You need to make sure you are taking a product that's free of contaminants.

On the label of the CBD products that you are considering make sure they contain the following: suggested serving size, servings per unit, and servings per package. The label information should tell you the product's "volume" so that you can determine how long it will last. A label stating "30 servings" means the product will last you for 30 days if it says that it is a once-a-day dosage. If twice a day then it will last you 15 days.

Preservation

Good CBD labels should provide cautions and instructions on preserving oil-based and other consumable product. Labels and/or packaging should state if the CBD oil needs to be stored in the refrigerator or just a cool place away from heat and light to preserve its medicinal potentacy. The label should also contain an expiration date, as all oil's go rancid over time.

Real Examples

Here are pictures of labels you'll see out on the market. Notice a couple of things about them.

One, no standards across brands. Two, notice how some manufacturers go the extra mile to make sure you are aware of everything in their product. Three, pay close attention to how other labels are very vague. Why is that?

Well, I can play the devil's advocate. The FDA hasn't set any standards, and since there aren't any standards, we'll just put what we think you need to know on the label and all is good. Or, we are a new company, and we don't have a good product label consultant to help us create medicinal product labels. We just put the results of the laboratory tests on the label. We understand what the label says, so should the consumer.

Hmmm. Sounds like a problem just waiting to happen.

At present, "CBD products are not produced under the guidance of good manufacturing practices (GMP) and are not subject to regulations governing labeling, purity, and reliability. In other words, currently, there is no guarantee of consistency between products, or even differing lots produced by the same manufacturer."

- Michael E. Schatman, PhD

Let's look at some suitable labels. These are making an attempt to show as much detail about the product as they can. I applaud that. Following that are some poor examples.

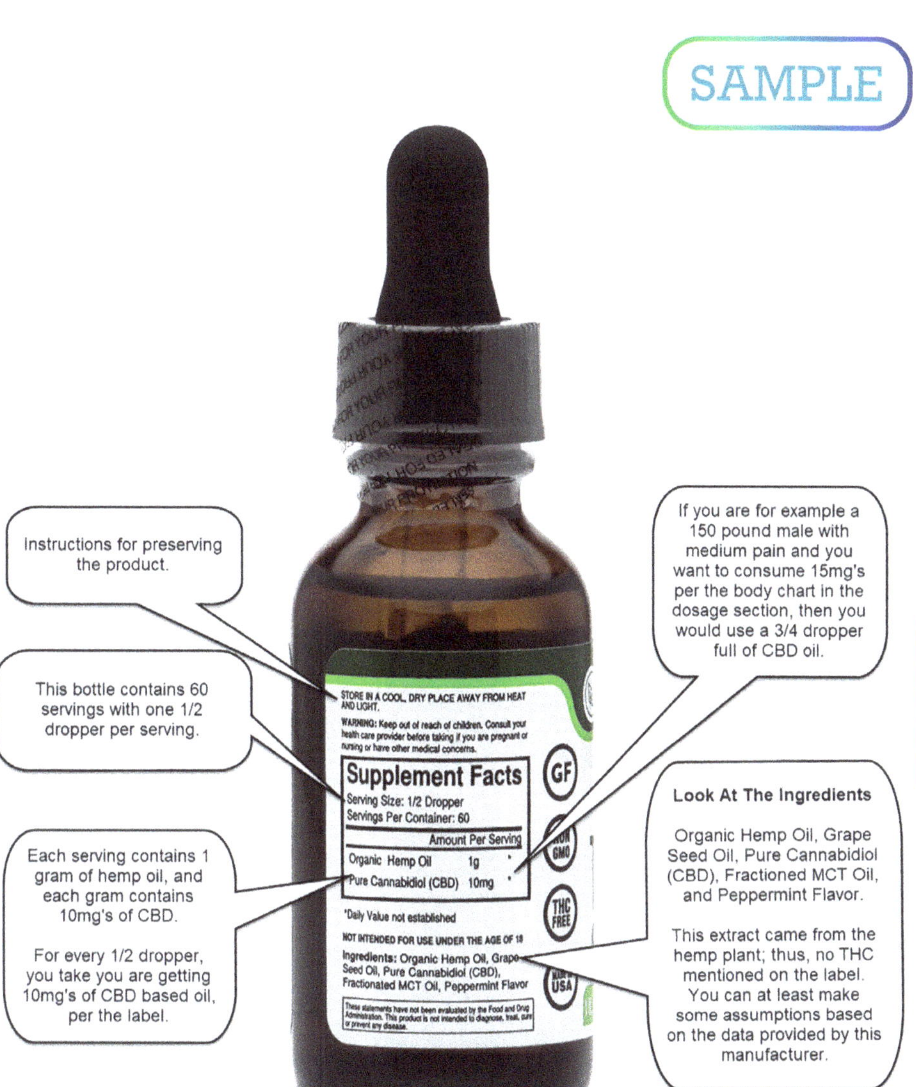

Figure 1 – Good label practices give customers peace of mind when purchasing. They feel they know what they are getting.

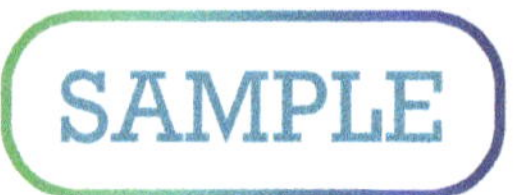

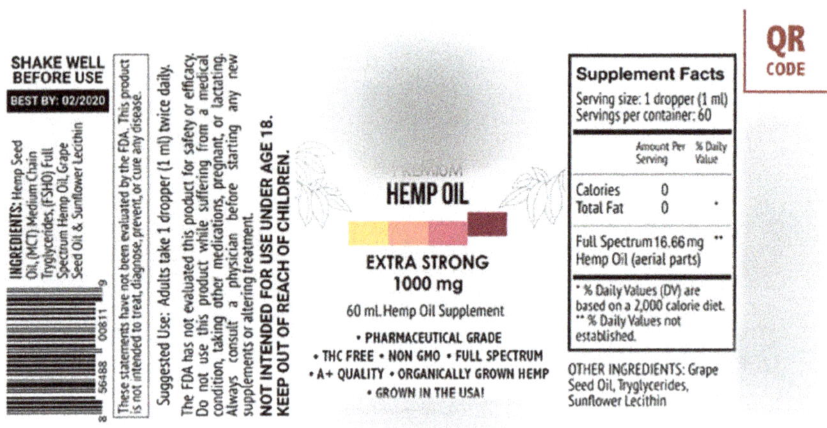

Figure 2 - Another well done label. You fully comprehend what and how much you are taking.

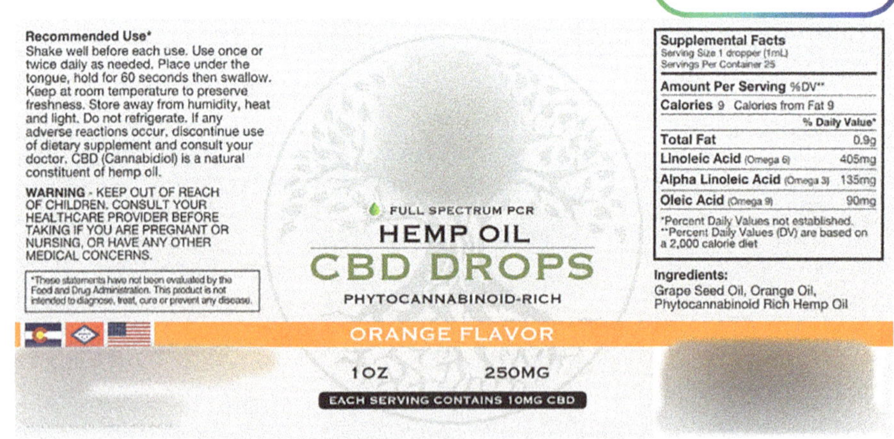

Figure 3 - Again, another well-organized label. Easy to read, easy to understand.

SOME NOT SO GOOD EXAMPLES OF CBD PRODUCT LABELS

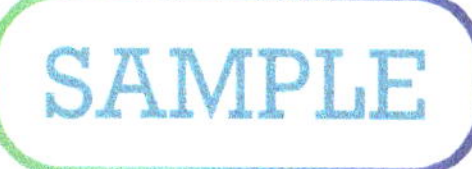

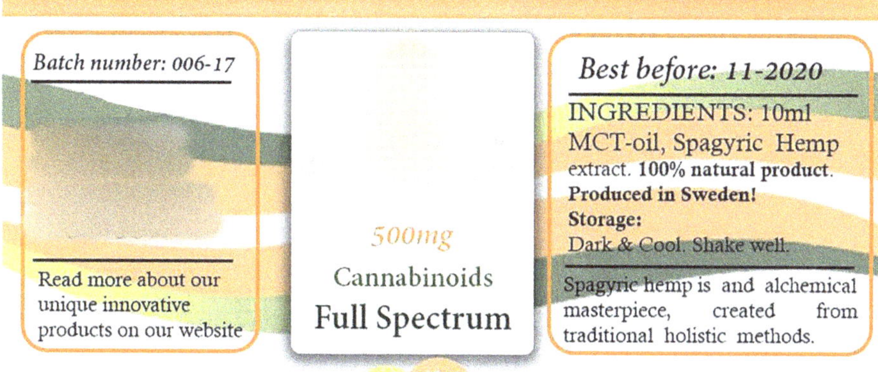

Figure 4 - I don't even know where to begin with this product.

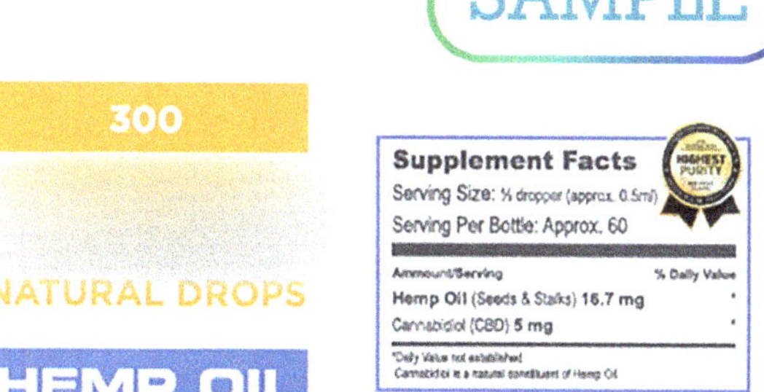

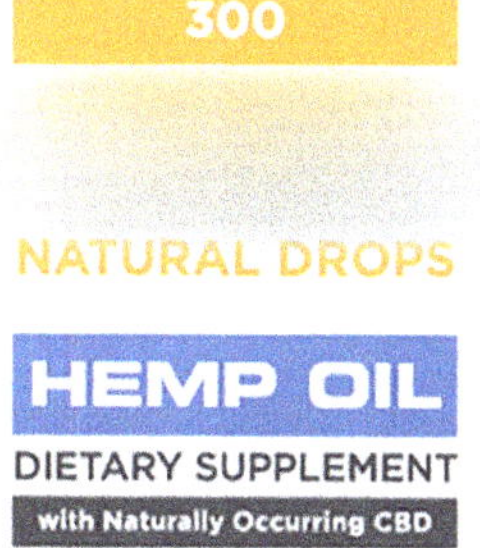

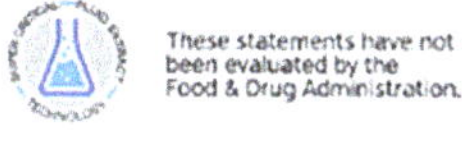

Use: Twice daily, or as needed.
Storage: In order to preserve freshness store away from excessive heat, light, and humidity.
Tamper Resistant: Use only if the safety seal is intact.
Warning: If pregnant or nursing, consult your physician before taking this or any other supplement.

KEEP OUT OF REACH OF CHILDREN

Elixinol CBD Hemp Oil is made from industrial hemp plants organically grown in Northern Europe. Our oil is cold-processed using CO2 super - critical fluid extraction resulting in a solvent free, pure extract.

This product is not intended to diagnose, treat, cure or prevent any disease.

These statements have not been evaluated by the Food & Drug Administration.

Supplement Facts

Serving Size: ½ dropper (approx. 0.5ml)

Serving Per Bottle: Approx. 60

Ammount/Serving	% Daily Value
Hemp Oil (Seeds & Stalks) 16.7 mg	•
Cannabidiol (CBD) 5 mg	•

*Daily Value not established.
Cannabidiol is a natural constituent of Hemp Oil.

OTHER INGREDIENTS:
Medium Chain Triglyceride Oil

Figure 5 - Honestly there is some information here, but truthfully this is a lazy job in labeling.

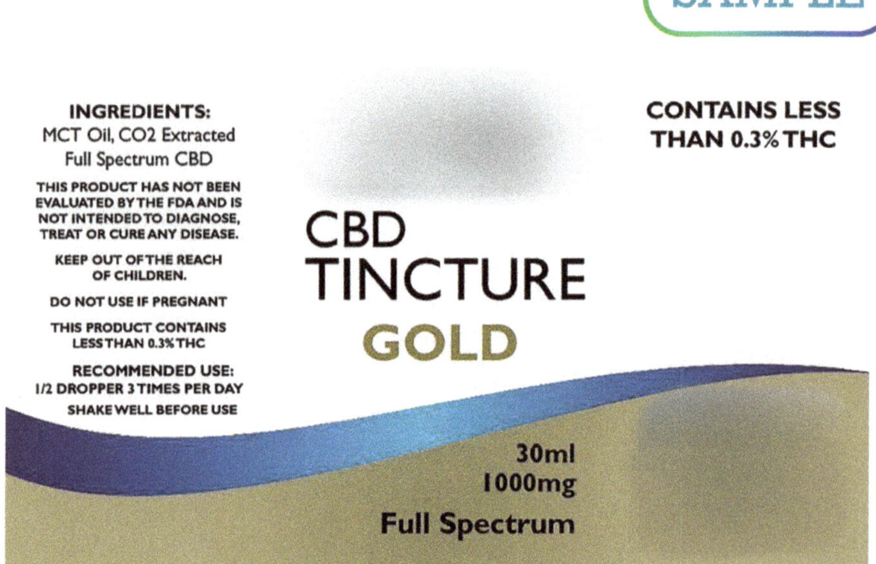

Figure 6 - Here is another example of "just get it to market, who cares what the label looks like." Its half assed.

GET TO KNOW WHAT YOU ARE LOOKING FOR WHEN IT COMES TO BUYING CBD PRODUCTS

Learn to understand the labeling of the products you are considering. Good quality manufacturers will post copies of their labels and their test results next to their products on their websites. If a manufacturer doesn't provide good quality product content information, purchase the product elsewhere. Trust me, speaking from experience, a bad product really is a waste of your time.

" LABELS SHOULD CONTAIN:

PRODUCT "VOLUME"
SUGGESTED SERVING SIZE
SERVINGS PER PACKAGE
AND SHOULD INCLUDE AN
EXPIRATION DATE "

CHAPTER 4

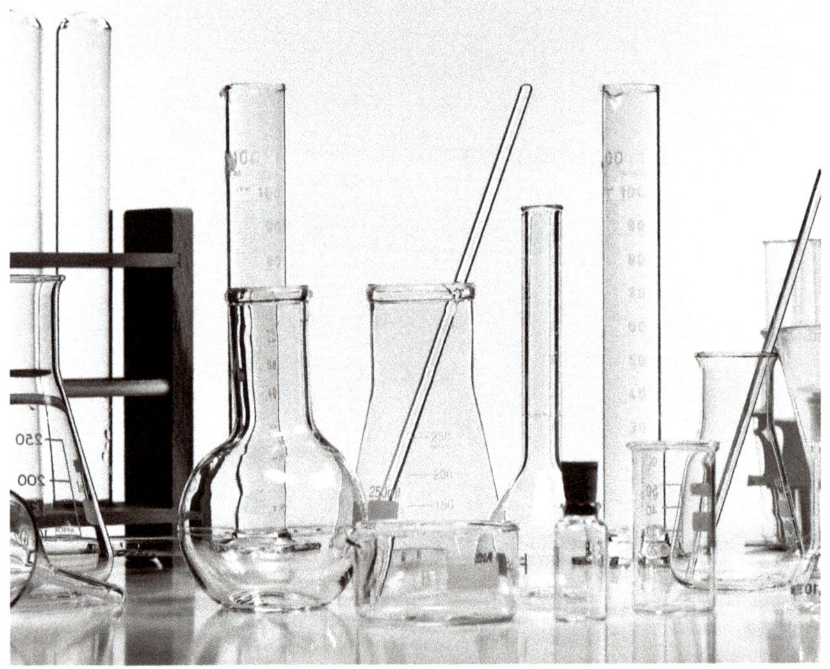

Testing

TESTING

INDEPENDENT THIRD PARTY TESTING

It's critical to have a neutral, independent laboratory testing the plant content and quality of a growers hemp product. From your perspective, this is incredibly important.

Today's market is a non-regulated state of commerce, and because of the lack of oversite by the FDA, it has essentially allowed manufacturers and distributors to glue medical-looking labels onto cute little bottles and then turn around and sell them as a cure-all.

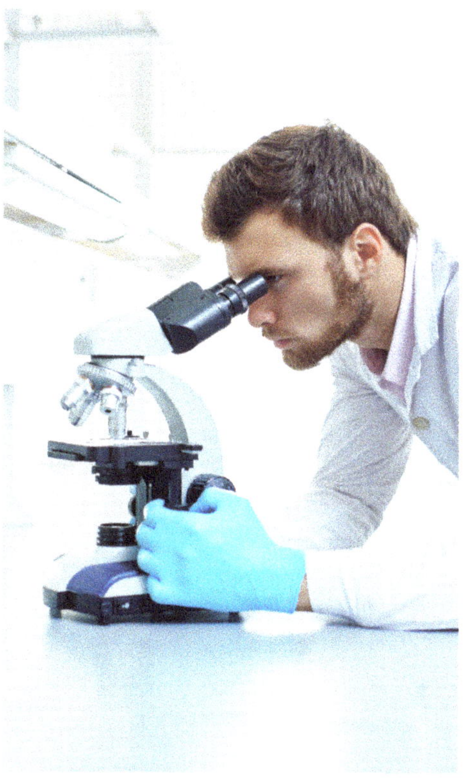

Hold on Charlie You Best Not Be Buyin That Junk!

Listen to me, don't you dare purchase any CBD or THC product over the Internet, without doing a little homework first, that's number one. Two, the same goes for purchasing from inside a store. You have my permission to buy online from any reputable source that tests their plant crop before processing and then tests again after the final product is ready to go market. Trust me there are 1,000's of things tested in between those two. Don't worry so much about that. That's product creation.

Over time oil goes rancid and potency diminishes. Hemp oil should be tested periodically, initially for impurities but to confirm efficacy as well. Testing safeguards you and establishes the amount of CBD advertised on the label, it tells you what's in the product, and that it has not exceeded the legal level of THC (0.3%). Proper testing and reporting show the company's transparency in its practice.

The Results of These Tests Can Be Found in the Form of a COA, or a Certificate of Analysis.

7 Ways to Manage Pain with CBD

The bottom line is, reputable manufacturers will test consistently and maintain a current COA or certificate of analysis and make it available to anyone who asks.

Kazmira, a CBD product manufacturer, gives us the best non-medical description of a "Certificate of Analysis" and why it's essential:

"A certificate of analysis (COA) is a lab report on the chemical make-up (e.g., contents) of a product. In the context of Industrial Hemp derived products, the COA shows the contents of the cannabinoids & other tested compounds such as heavy metals, etc. COA's are used to verify that the contents of the product are matched to the advertised or marketed product. These reports are important for verifying that hemp extracts have less than .3% THC, as determined by the definition of Industrial Hemp in the law." - kazmira-llc.com

Look for Companies That are Transparent With Their Internal Processes

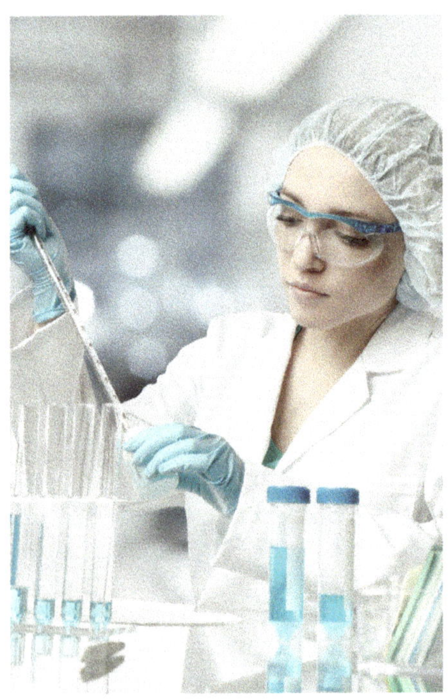

With hemp products and CBD oil, in particular, becoming more and more popular by the day, it's crucial for companies who are publicly consumed brands to establish themselves as reliable and reputable.

Now that you know what a good quality CBD oil is capable of doing in a person's body in terms of relief from chronic pain if a company/brand isn't confident enough to have their products tested by an independent laboratory, their products aren't worth your hard-earned money being spent on them.

I will stand firm on this platform and say this: that only Independent third-party lab test results should be used on what is "labeled and presented" for public consumption. The manufacturers internal testing facility results should not be used on packaging, labeling, or in advertisements.

Otherwise, you have no assurance of the claims being made about the amount, the quality, or the strength of the CBD oil/product. The standard - high CBD, low THC, no harmful impurities, period.

Brands that are trying to distinguish themselves as trustworthy will always provide high-resolution images of their label, of recent independent lab results, and they should be made available to download as a pdf so you can print them.

Some now provide those on their website, while others include them in the packaging or both. If there is a toll-free number to call on the label or website chances are they are making every effort to be a legitimate company providing some customer service. Call them and ask them to help you if you're having trouble finding the lab results. You want to see them. Did you read that clearly? You want to see them!

Things to look for in a COA

- Potency Analysis
- Heavy Metal Analysis
- Pesticide Analysis
- Terpene Profiles

Good quality "THC-Free CBD oil" and "broad spectrum hemp oils" should first and foremost have high levels of CBD. Full spectrum should have other cannabinoids such as CBG or CBN, but no detectable levels of THC. High-quality full spectrum hemp extracts should have many varieties of cannabinoids, and some might include trace amounts of THC. As long as the THC weight percent (%) is below 0.3%, they are within the legal limits allowed by the federal government. Remember that's not enough to make you feel high.

"Eighty-four products were purchased and analyzed (from 31 companies). Median labeled concentration was 15.00 mg/mL. With respect to CBD, 42.85% of products were underlabeled, 26.19% were overlabeled, and 30.95% were accurately labeled."

- Study published in JAMA by researchers at Johns Hopkins School of Medicine and University of Pennsylvania Perelman School of Medicine

This next section is going to be a little bit technical. The incredible scientists and our good friends at G2 Analytical put together this article on how to read the "Lab Results" or the "Certificate of Analysis" of a CBD manufacturers product.

I've broken it down into small chunks of information so that you can digest little bits at a time. If you're the technical type, you're going to love reading this. For you, non-techies do your best to muddle through. I'm sorry but required reading.

HOW TO READ
THE
LAB RESULTS

Lab reports can be confusing. Often referred to as Certificates of Analysis, these reports contain information about the potency of the product. They may also include results for various contamination testing that is performed. With numbers, percentages, and graphs, the amount of information the labs are trying to convey can feel overwhelming. Lab report formats vary; however, they should contain some basic components, and you should know how to read them.

Apples-to-Apples: As simple as it seems, the most important thing to look for is the product information. All lab reports should clearly state the name of the product that is tested. Make sure the name of the product tested is the exact same as the label item you are buying. Also, make sure the batch number of the product you are buying matches the batch number tested. Some products do not use batch numbers, and that makes verifying test results more challenging. Many lab reports also have a product description, and date received and tested that also aid in the validation of lab reports.

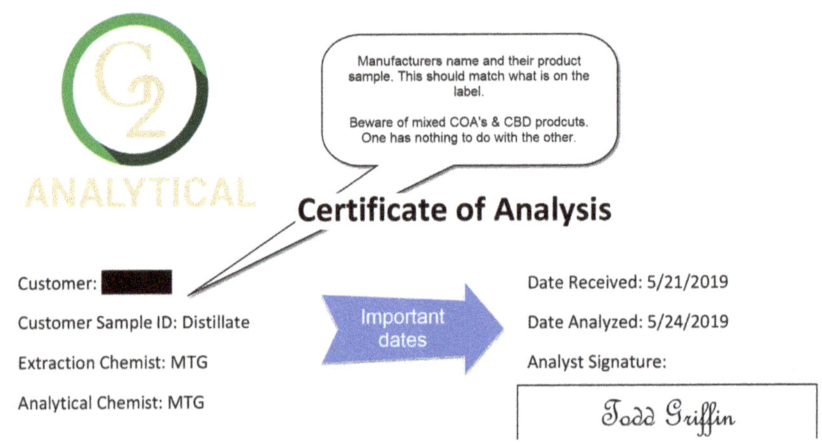

What's Your Number?

Next, we look at what's in the reports. The most common test is potency. The potency is simply the amount of active ingredient (cannabinoids) that are in the sample. This is often referred to as a cannabinoid panel since labs will test for multiple cannabinoids simultaneously.

TESTING

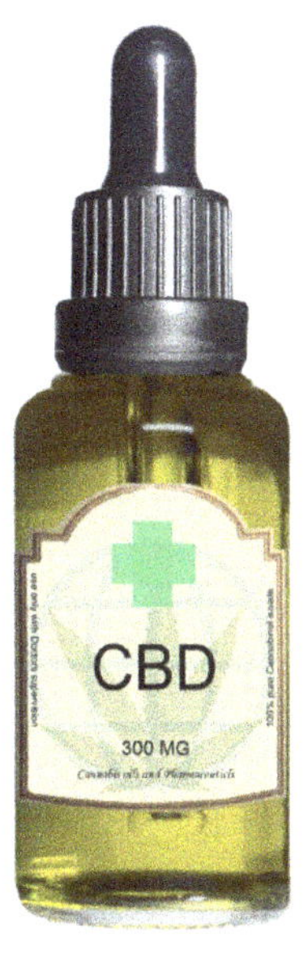

Most labs screen between 3-11 different cannabinoids. CBD and THC are the major cannabinoids of interest because they occur in the highest levels. For tinctures and other liquid products, the results are listed as mass, typically milligrams, of the cannabinoid per volume, typically milliliters.

However, products are usually labeled with the milligrams of cannabinoid in the entire bottle. For example, a 1 fluid ounce (~30 mL) bottle of CBD oil may be labeled as 300 mg. This would represent a concentration of 10 mg CBD per 1 mL of sample.

A 30mL bottle / 300mg = 10mg per serving.

Other dosage forms may report mass percent. This is simply the mass (typically grams) of the cannabinoid divided by the total mass of product (typically grams) and reported as a percentage.

Therefore, an 18% CBD flower, would contain 180 milligrams of CBD for every gram of flower. In order to be considered hemp, the THC concentration cannot be more than 0.3%. Thus, we need the mass percent to be less than 0.3% which is 0.3 milligram per gram of flower (or ~0.34 milligram per milliliter of oil).

Cannabinoid Profile	Limits of Quantification (LOQ)		Results	
	mg/mL	Mass Percent	mg/mL	Mass Percent
Cannabidiolic Acid (CBDA)	2.0	0.22%	ND*	-
Cannabidiol (CBD)	2.0	0.22%	1.63	0.17
Δ9-Tetrahydrocannabidol (THC)	2.0	0.22%	<LOQ**	-

Mass Analyzed: 106.2 mg

Average mass of CBD: 81.27 mg

Mass Percent of CBD in Distillate: 76.5%

Comments:

Distillate was dissolved in 50.00 mL of MCT oil for analysis.

* CBDA was not detected.

** THC was detected but was less than the limit of quantification listed above.

Beware of the Terms "Total CBD" and "Total THC"

Another critical piece of information you should be aware of is the terms "total CBD" and "total THC."

Cannabis naturally makes acidic versions of the cannabinoids (e.g., CBDA or THCA). It is only through heating that CBDA and THCA are converted to their "active" forms. Since CBDA and THCA are not metabolized in the human body, they remain in their original, acidic form.

Only certain lab techniques can differentiate between the acidic forms and active forms. Therefore, some labs report "total CBD" and/or "total THC," and those numbers are the combination of the acid and active forms.

While they may have some similar effects, they are certainly not going to interact with the endocannabinoid system in the same manner as their active forms. For products meant to be consumed orally or topically, consumers should look for lab reports that differentiate between the acids and active forms.

Finally, full spectrum products should contain multiple cannabinoids. The entourage effect relies on a mixture of cannabinoids to enhance the efficacy of the cannabinoids. Therefore, if your product is labeled as full spectrum, but the lab report only shows CBD, the product is either made from an isolate (a single cannabinoid) or the lab did not test for the minor cannabinoids.

Contaminants

Contamination from pesticide, heavy metals, residual solvents, toxin, and pathogen testing is also very important for consumers. Since hemp readily absorbs contaminants from the soil and hemp products are often derived from contracts or extracts, pesticide and heavy metals should be tested.

Handling, storing, and processing the hemp can lead to further contamination. Results are usually presented in a "pass/fail" manner. Limits are set at the action levels determined by government regulation, and if a contaminant is detected above that limit, it is flagged. So, if you have a test report with all "not detected" that means that these contaminants were not present. If you have questions about these lab reports, just ask for help.

Retailers should be very conversant in the details of the lab reports from their vendors. This is why it is important to develop a relationship with the dispensary or store. Many vendors and labs provide in-service training to store employees to help them understand the product and all testing.

Independent testing labs are also usually very eager to help consumers navigate through test results. At the end of the day, you must be satisfied with the results of any lab tests, and you deserve total confidence in the product you consume.

Canabinoid Potency Analysis

Substance	Weight (%)	mg/g
THCa	0.006	0.060
D9-THC	0.201	2.010
D8-THC	<LOQ*	<LOQ*
THCV	0.002	0.020
THCVa	<LOQ*	<LOQ*
TOTAL THC	0.209	2.090
CBDa	0.406	4.060
CBD	5.620	56.20
CBDV	0.036	0.360
CBDVa	ND*	ND*
TOTAL CBD	6.062	60.62
CBN	0.009	0.090
CBG	0.172	1.720
CBGa	0.036	0.360
CBC	0.222	2.220
TOTAL CANNABINOIDS	6.501	65.01

* CBDa Not Detected

** THC was detected but was less than the "limit of quantification" listed above

Pay close attention to these "terms & abbreviations," you will see them repeatedly to varying levels.

Listed are just as a handful of examples. There are many more.

TESTING

Terpenes

Another popular test shows the terpene profiles. Terpenes are known for their unique and strong odor. While the profiles were originally thought to be for user preference (like the bouquet of wines), there is ongoing research about potential health benefits. Therefore, many lab reports lists which terpenes are present.

There are more than 100 terpenes in just one Flower (plant). Here are some of the most well known terpenes in use now. Most of which you'll find in legal cannabis products.

Terpene Name	Aroma	Properties	Common Uses
Bisabolol	floral	anti-inflammatory anti-irritant anti-microbial	cancer, skin lesion
Borneol	mint	anti-inflammatory antinociceptive	eyesight, pain relief
Camphene	fir needles musky earth	anti-oxidant	skin lesion cardiovascular diseases
Caryophyllene	spicy	anti-bacterial anti-inflammatory anti-fungal	insomnia, muscle spasms pain relief
Delta 3 Carene	pine rosemary	anti-inflammatory	bone stimulant memory
Eucalyptol	mint	anti-bacterial anti-fungal	alzheimer's pain Relief
Geraniol	peach rose grass	anti-cancer anti-oxidant neuroprotectant	cancer, pain relief
Humulene	earthy	anti-bacterial anti-inflammatory anti-tumor effects	appetite suppression cancer,infections pain relieft
Limonene	bitter citrus	anti-anxiety anti-cancer	digestion, gallstones liver detoxification weight loss, sleep aid
Linalool	floral	anti-anxiety anti-epileptic anti-psychotic pain killing	depression, convulsions insomnia, pain relief

Myrcene	citrus cloves	relaxing, sedating	inflammation, insomnia spasms, pain
Pinene	pine	anti-depressant anti-inflammatory anti-microbial	asthma, bronchitis cancer, depression memory, mental alertness
Phytol	balsamic floral	anti-insomnia immunosuppressant	reduce itching sleep aid wound healing
Terpinolene	smoky woody	anti-bacterial anti-fungal anti-insomnia antiseptic	cancer, heart disease sleep aid
Trans-nerolidol	citrus rose	anti-cancer anti-microbial anti-oxidant, anti-parasitic	relaxing skin lesion
Valencene	sweet citrus	anti-inflammatory anti-melanogenesis antiallergic	memory skin lesion

Following are a few examples of what a COA "Certificate of Analysis" looks like. Notice as you did in the labels section, from testing facility to state to federal level, there are no standards.

These are not recomendations! Please do not purchase these samples, they have not been properly vetted to make sure they meet all of the standards that I'm talking about in this book.

These are for illustrative purposes only.

NOTE:
If you have difficulty reading these condensed COA and label examples, please email me or visit my website for better quality examples. Getting these COA's to be high quality for print was not an easy task. If you feel I've missed something and should include it in this book, let me know. If I use it, I'll send you a free updated copy of the book for taking the effort.
Email: inforequest@thecbdwriter.com
Website: https://thecbdwriter.com

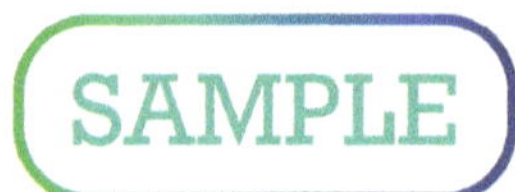

LABORATORY CANNABINOID PROFILE CERTIFICATE OF ANALYSIS	Extraction Date:09-Oct-18
	Analysis Date/Time:09-Oct-18, 12:45:03

CUSTOMER INFORMATION		SAMPLE DETAILS	
Company:		Sample Name	CBD Full Spectrum Oil 500mg
Contact Person:		Sample Number	11488, 11489
Contact Email:		Sample Information	500mg
Contact phone:			Average of 2 replicates

Substance Potency Analysis

CANNABINOID	Mg. PER GRAM	TOTAL Mg. IN A	15	GRAM PACKAGE (as reported by client)
CBD MAXIMUM *	38.85	582.68		
THC MAXIMUM *	0.20	3.00		
CBDA	ND[1]	ND[1]		
CBG	0.12	1.79		
CBD	38.85	582.68		
CBN	ND[1]	ND[1]		
THC	0.20	3.00		
CBC	0.39	5.90		
THCA	ND[1]	ND[1]		

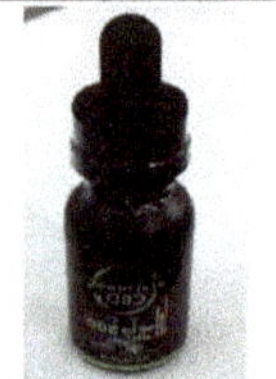

Substance Distribution Analysis

COLOR CODE	CANNABINOID	% BY WEIGHT	Distribution
	CBDA	ND[1]	ND[1]
	CBG	0.01	0.30%
	CBD	3.88	98.20%
	CBN	ND[1]	ND[1]
	THC	0.02	0.51%
	CBC	0.04	0.99%
	THCA	ND[1]	ND[1]

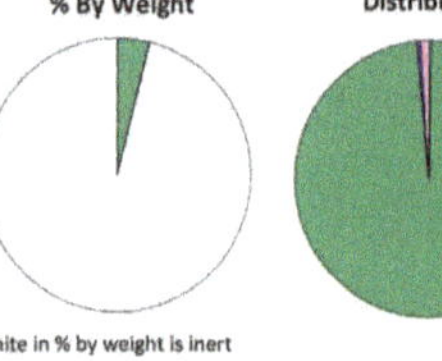
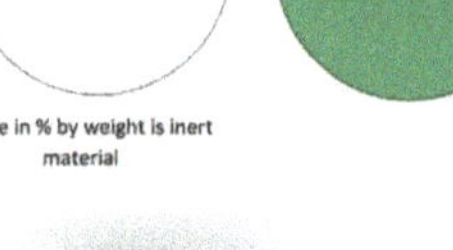

* All cannabinoids in their acid forms (ending in "A") are convertible to their non-acid forms via a decarboxylation process (heating). The THC and CBD maximum values reported above are the maximum theoretical amounts of THC and CBD the tested product would have if it were fully decarboxylated.

Maximum % THC values exceeding three-tenths of one percent (0.3%) on a dry weight basis do not qualify as industrial hemp

Maximum % THC Value for this sample is: 0.02 %

[1] Cannabinoid not detected (ND).

[2] Cannabinoid detected below Limit of Quantitation (LOQ).

This test report may not be duplicated, except in full with permission from   . All testing reports represent a strict confidentiality agreement between   and the client listed on the report. No discussion of certificates of analysis will be permitted except with authorized parties of the client indicated on the certificate of analysis.

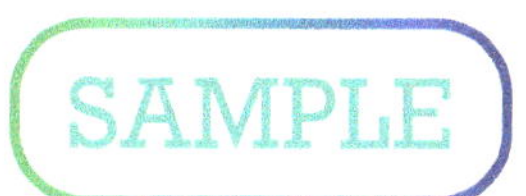

Certificate of Analysis

CBD Oil 240mg
Matrix: Oil

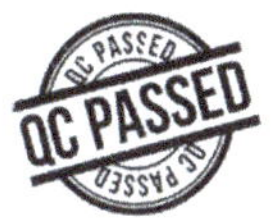

SAMPLE: D804023-01
Harvest/Lot ID: BB-18-01
Batch#: BB-18-01; Batch Size:N/A
Ordered: 04/12/2018; Sampled: N/A
Completed: 04/26/2018; Expires: 04/26/2019
Sampling Method: Client Method

Image

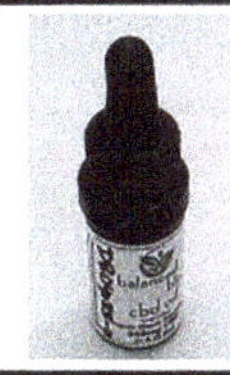

Pesticides – NT
Microbials- NT
Mycotoxins – NT
Heavy Metals - NT
Terpenes - Page 2
Residual Solvents – NT
Filth – NT
Water Activity – NT
Moisture – NT

Cannabinoids

Analyte	Weight (%)	mg/g	RPD%
THCa	0.006	0.060	
D9-THC	0.209	2.090	
D8-THC	<LOQ	<LOQ	
THCV	0.008	0.080	
THCVa	<LOQ	<LOQ	
TOTAL THC	**0.214**	**2.143**	
CBDa	0.427	4.270	
CBD	5.320	53.20	
CBDV	0.033	0.330	
CBDVa	<LOQ	<LOQ	
TOTAL CBD	**5.694**	**56.945**	
CBN	0.015	0.150	
CBG	0.165	1.650	
CBGa	0.023	0.230	
CBC	0.262	2.620	
TOTAL CANNABINOIDS	**6.468**	**64.680**	

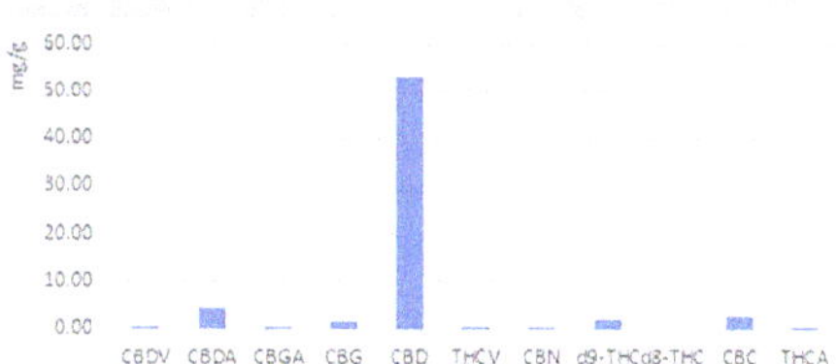

State License # N/A

7 Ways to Manage Pain with CBD

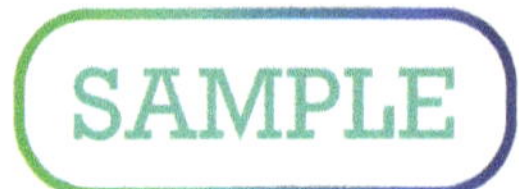

CERTIFICATE OF ANALYSIS

Elektra

Batch ID:	A07R	Test ID:	3433851.010
Reported:	25-Oct-2018	Method:	TM01
Type:	Plant		
Test:	Potency		

CANNABINOID PROFILE

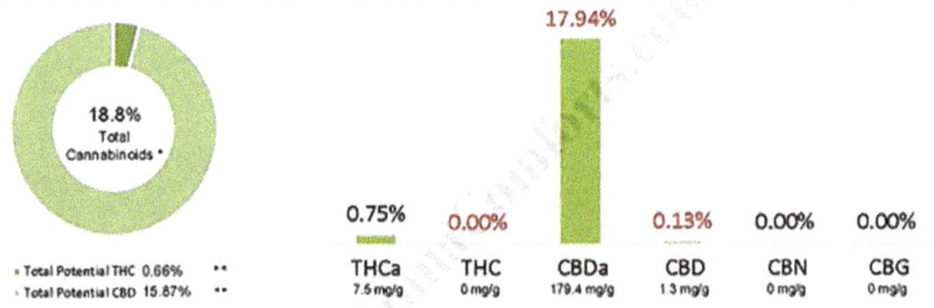

* Total Cannabinoids result reflects the absolute sum of all cannabinoids detected.
** Total Potential THC/CBD is calculated using the following formulas to take into account the loss of a carboxyl group during decarboxylation step.
Total THC = THC + (THCa *0.877) and Total CBD = CBD + (CBDa *0.877)
% = % (w/w) = Percent (Weight of Analyte / Weight of Product)

NOTES
Free from visual mold, mildew, and foreign matter.

FINAL APPROVAL

PREPARED BY / DATE

APPROVED BY / DATE

Testing results are based solely upon the sample submitted to , condition it was received. ,
, warrants that all analytical work is conducted professionally in accordance with all applicable standard laboratory practices using
validated methods. Data was generated using an unbroken chain of comparison to NIST traceable Reference Standards and Certified
Reference Materials. This report may not be reproduced, except in full, without the written approval of

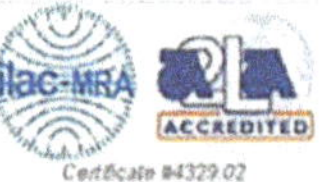

Certificate #4329.02

"FAMILIARIZE YOURSELF WITH THE ANALYSIS OF POTENCY, HEAVY METALS, PESTICIDES, AND TERPENE PROFILES."

CHAPTER 5

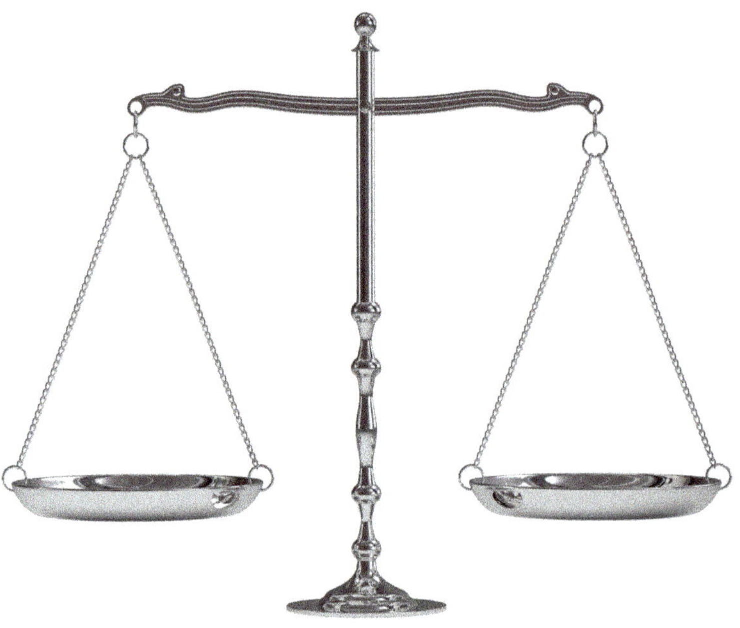

Is It Legal?

IS IT LEGAL?

This summary of hemp legalality and following state list is by Bill Hines writing for the Matador Network. As he puts it:

"The 2018 Farm Bill legalized a lot of CBD, but not all of it. Most importantly, it redefined what hemp and hemp products are by federal law. Hemp is legally defined as a cannabis plant or part of the cannabis plant that has a THC concentration "of not more than 0.3 percent on a dry weight basis. That's not enough to get you high, and CBD with less than 0.3 percent THC is also not strong enough to make you fail a drug test."

Note: Some would say "CBD with less than (0.3%) THC is not strong enough to make you fail a drug test," this author says "caveat emptor," "buyer beware." The jury is still out.

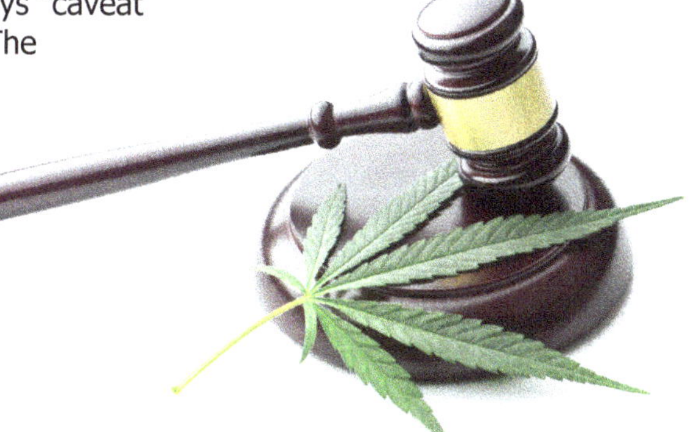

"If the THC concentration is higher, however, then it's classified as a Schedule I drug under the Controlled Substances Act.

That means the US Drug Enforcement Administration believes it has "no currently accepted medical use and a high potential for abuse."

Cannabis Laws by State CBD and CBD product/oil legality

"Thanks to the 2018 Farm Bill, hemp-derived CBD is federally allowed in every state, and licensed companies are allowed to commercially distribute CBD products across state lines. The bill allows states to create more strict laws than the federal legislation, however, meaning states can ban CBD specifically."

As far as we are concerned, that's all we care about. CBD products being shipped to all 50 states.

These are the specific laws for each state as of 2019.

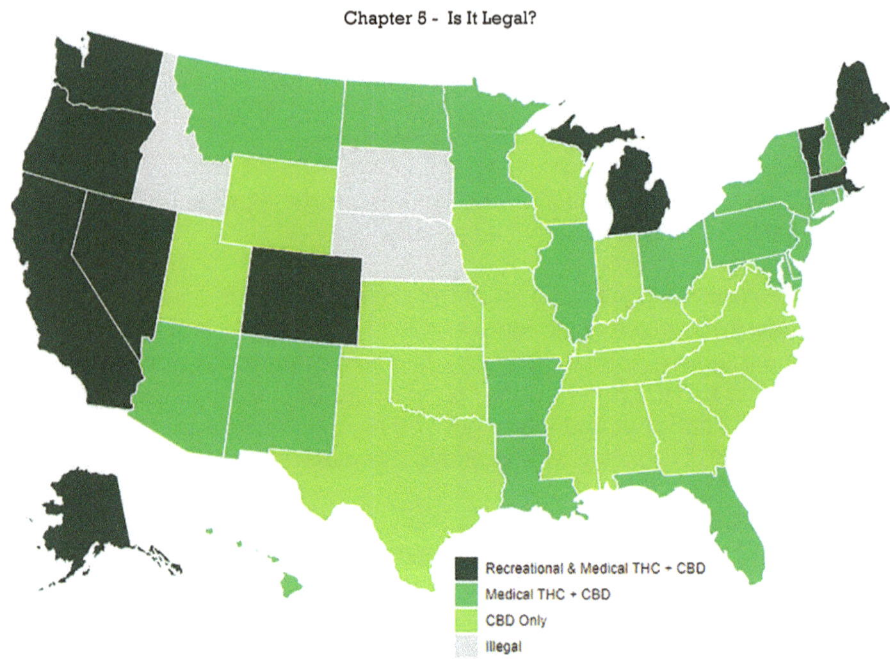

Source: **NORML** (The National Organization for Reform of Marijuana Laws) and, for states with legal medical and recreational marijuana, from a CR analysis of state policies. The legality of shipping CBD across state lines is ambiguous. This information is for educational purposes and is not legal advice. Updated as of April 11, 2019.

✓ Alabama: Legal under 2018 Farm Bill rules.

✓ Alaska: Both hemp- and cannabis -derived CBD produced in the state is legal under the state's recreational cannabis laws. Any CBD product created from cannabis or made by a federally unlicensed grower is federally illegal and cannot be shipped across state lines.

✓ Arizona: Legal under 2018 Farm Bill rules.

✓ Arkansas: Legal under 2018 Farm Bill rules.

✓ California: Both hemp- and cannabis -derived CBD produced in the state is legal under the state's recreational cannabis laws. Any CBD product created from cannabis or made by a federally unlicensed grower is federally illegal and cannot be shipped across state lines.

✓ Colorado: Both hemp- and cannabis -derived CBD produced in the state is legal under the state's recreational cannabis laws. Any CBD product created from cannabis or made by a federally unlicensed grower is federally illegal and cannot be shipped across state lines.

✓ Connecticut: Legal under 2018 Farm Bill rules.

✓ Delaware: Legal under 2018 Farm Bill rules.

✓ Florida: Legal under 2018 Farm Bill rules.

✓ Georgia: Legal under 2018 Farm Bill rules.

✓ Hawaii: Legal under 2018 Farm Bill rules.

✓ Idaho: Only CBD products with 0.0 percent THC.

✓ Illinois: Legal under 2018 Farm Bill rules.

✓ Indiana: Legal under 2018 Farm Bill rules.

✓ Iowa: Legal under 2018 Farm Bill rules.

✓ Kansas: Legal under 2018 Farm Bill rules.

✓ Kentucky: Legal under 2018 Farm Bill rules.

✓ Louisiana: Legal under 2018 Farm Bill rules.

- ✓ Maine: Both hemp- and cannabis-derived CBD produced in the state is legal under the state's recreational cannabis laws. Any CBD product created from cannabis or made by a federally unlicensed grower is federally illegal and cannot be shipped across state lines.
- ✓ Maryland: Legal under 2018 Farm Bill rules.
- ✓ Massachusetts Both hemp- and cannabis-derived CBD produced in the state is legal under the state's recreational cannabis laws. Any CBD product created from cannabis or made by a federally unlicensed grower is federally illegal and cannot be shipped across state lines.
- ✓ Michigan: Both hemp- and cannabis-derived CBD produced in the state is legal under the state's recreational cannabis laws. Any CBD product created from cannabis or made by a federally unlicensed grower is federally illegal and cannot be shipped across state lines.
- ✓ Minnesota: Legal under 2018 Farm Bill rules.
- ✓ Mississippi: Legal under 2018 Farm Bill rules.
- ✓ Missouri: Legal under 2018 Farm Bill rules.
- ✓ Montana: Legal under 2018 Farm Bill rules.
- ✓ Nebraska: All CBD is illegal and anyone selling CBD can be prosecuted.
- ✓ Nevada: Both hemp- and cannabis-derived CBD produced in the state is legal under the state's recreational cannabis laws. Any CBD product created from cannabis or made by a federally unlicensed grower is federally illegal and cannot be shipped across state lines.
- ✓ New Hampshire: Legal under 2018 Farm Bill rules.
- ✓ New Jersey: Legal under 2018 Farm Bill rules.
- ✓ New Mexico: Legal under 2018 Farm Bill rules.
- ✓ New York: Legal under 2018 Farm Bill rules.
- ✓ North Carolina: Legal under 2018 Farm Bill rules.
- ✓ North Dakota: Legal under 2018 Farm Bill rules.
- ✓ Ohio: Legal under 2018 Farm Bill rules.
- ✓ Oklahoma: Legal under 2018 Farm Bill rules.
- ✓ Oregon: Both hemp- and cannabis-derived CBD produced in the state is legal under the state's recreational cannabis laws. Any CBD product created from cannabis or made by a federally unlicensed grower is federally illegal and cannot be shipped across state lines.
- ✓ Pennsylvania: Legal under 2018 Farm Bill rules.
- ✓ Rhode Island: Legal under 2018 Farm Bill rules.
- ✓ South Carolina: Legal under 2018 Farm Bill rules.
- ✓ South Dakota: All CBD is illegal and anyone selling CBD can be prosecuted.
- ✓ Tennessee: Legal under 2018 Farm Bill rules.
- ✓ Texas: Legal under 2018 Farm Bill rules.
- ✓ Utah: Legal under 2018 Farm Bill rules.
- ✓ Vermont: Both hemp- and cannabis-derived CBD produced in the state is legal under the state's recreational cannabis laws. Any CBD product created from cannabis or made by a federally unlicensed grower is federally illegal and cannot be shipped across state lines.
- ✓ Virginia: Legal under 2018 Farm Bill rules.
- ✓ Washington: Both hemp- and cannabis-derived CBD produced in the state is legal under the state's recreational cannabis laws. Any CBD product created from cannabis or made by a federally unlicensed grower is federally illegal and cannot be shipped across state lines.
- ✓ West Virginia: Legal under 2018 Farm Bill rules.
- ✓ Wisconsin: Legal under 2018 Farm Bill rules.
- ✓ Wyoming: Legal under 2018 Farm Bill rules.

SUMMARY

CBD products are becoming extremely popular among all ages. This trend is being fueled by the ever-growing amount of studies demonstrating CBD's therapeutic potential.

The purpose of this book is to give you multiple methods of using CBD to find relief from your pain. This book only scratches the surface in regards to using CBD, but it is more than enough to get you started and pointed into the right direction. What you do from here at this moment in your life now is a whole new journey for you in finding relief from pain. Big pharma, of course, will be unhappy about losing money, but I promise you I won't be losing any sleep.

Has this book impacted your life, please send me a video or an email to itworks@thecbdwriter.com. I would love to hear your story. Not only that, if you share your account with us, we may use it in future book updates and on our website. With your permission, of course.

Also, I am available for speaking engagements. Please email my staff for more information.

I wish you the best, and I look forward to hearing from you.

APPENDIX

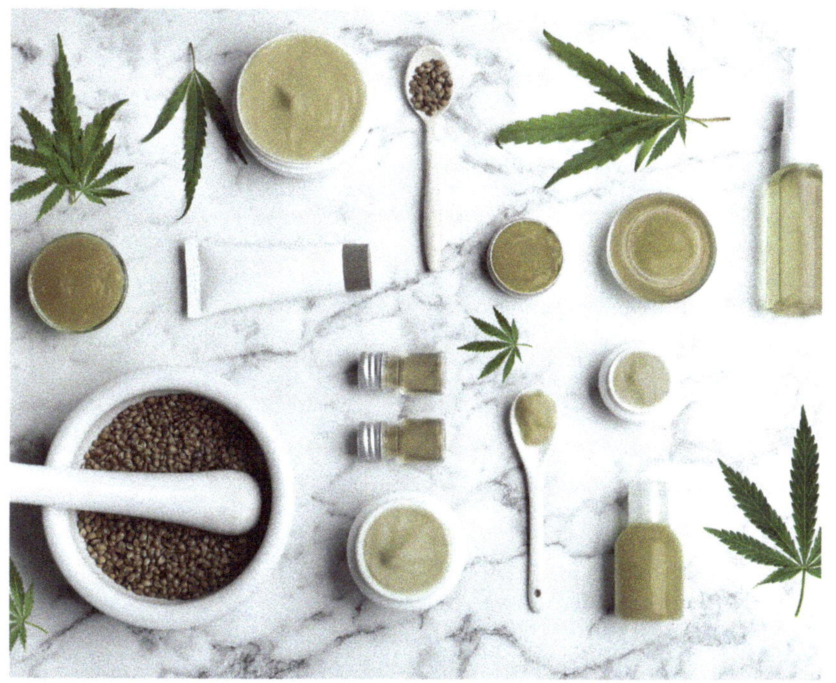

Studies & Additional Information

STUDIES

These following links are just the beginning of what is available in regards to research using Cannabis/Hemp. Here starts the beginning of your journey to learn more.

Project CBD: They have enough to keep your research habits fed for a couple of years. Their pain page has more information than most informational websites. They actively are trying to educate consumers.

They have a good depth of quality medical related material dealing with pain and using cannabis.
https://www.projectcbd.org/cbd-for/pain

The Effects of CBD on the Human Body, as explained by a Doctor
http://bit.ly/effects-of-cbd

Understanding the Endocannabinoid System - NIDA/NIH
http://bit.ly/e-c-s

Cannabinoid Delivery Systems for Pain and Inflammation Treatment
http://bit.ly/Pain-and-Inflammation

CBD: How It Works
http://bit.ly/CBD-How-It-Works

A double-blind, randomized, placebo-controlled, parallel group study of THC/CBD spray in peripheral neuropathic pain treatment
http://bit.ly/CBD-neuro-pain

Medical Marijuana: The State of the Science
http://bit.ly/medical-marijuana-science

Repeated CBD Doses Required for Effective Pain Relief
http://bit.ly/CBD-Pain-Relief

Cannabis Use in Patients with Fibromyalgia: Effect on Symptoms Relief and Health-Related Quality of Life
http://bit.ly/Fibromyalgia-Relief

Personal experience and attitudes of pain medicine specialists in Israel regarding the medical use of cannabis for chronic pain
http://bit.ly/cannabis-for-chronic-pain

A Cross-Sectional Study of Cannabidiol Users
http://bit.ly/study-of-cbd-users

REFERENCES

Pg: ii CNN: For doctors, more opioid prescriptions bring more money
URL: http://bit.ly/Opioid-Payments

Pg. iii: Web MD: "Pain Classifications and Causes: Nerve Pain, Muscle Pain, and More"
URL: http://bit.ly/Pain-Types

Pg. iv: Dr. David Allen: The Discovery of the Endocannabinoid System
URL: http://bit.ly/Dr-David-Allen

Pg. iv: Lester Grinspoon, MD Biography
Testimony before the Crime Subcommittee of the Judiciary Committee in the US House of Representatives, October 1, 1997

Pg. v: Physicians Grade: "Physicians Speak About Cannabidiol"
URL: http://bit.ly/CBD-Physicians

Pg v: CNN: WEED: A Dr. Sanjay Gupta Investigation. Aired August 11, 2013
URL: http://bit.ly/Dr-Gupta-Weed

Pg. vi: Health.com: 7 Surprising Ways People Are Using CBD Oil-and What Doctors Really Think About It
URL: http://bit.ly/7-Ways-CBD-Oil

Pg. vi: British Journal of Clinical Pharmacology: "Cannabinoids for treatment of chronic non-cancer pain; a systematic review of randomized trials"
URL: http://bit.ly/Random-Trials

Pg. 4: Dr. Sanjay Gupta: "Cannabis Can Be a Gateway to Recovery"
URL: http://bit.ly/Cannabis-Recovery

Pg. 4: Dr. Sanjay Gupta Marijuana Research Mention.
URL: http://bit.ly/Gupta-Research

Pg. 6: What is CBD: "HOW DOES CBD WORK"
URL: http://bit.ly/How-CBD-Works

Pg. 6: Patient survey: Cannabis in the treatment of age-related pain.
URL: http://bit.ly/Age-Related-Pain

Pg. 10: CBDNewsFeed.com: 10 High-Profile Celebrities Who Use CBD
URL: http://bit.ly/CBD-Celebrities

Pg. 17: Medical Marijuana: The State of the Science
URL: http://bit.ly/MMJ-Science

7 Ways to Manage Pain with CBD

REFERENCES

Pg. 18: Molecules (Basel, Switzerland): "Cannabinoid Delivery Systems for Pain and Inflammation Treatment"
URL: http://bit.ly/Pain-and-Inflammation

Pg. 20: Wikipedia: Oral administration
URL: http://bit.ly/Oral-Admin

Pg: 24: European Journal of Pharmacology: "An entourage effect: inactive endogenous fatty acid glycerol esters enhance 2-arachidonoyl-glycerol cannabinoid activity"
URL: http://bit.ly/Entourage-Effect

Pg: 27: Wikipedia: Sublingual administration
URL: http://bit.ly/CBD-Sublingual

Pg. 34: Medscape Neurology News: Repeated CBD Doses Required for Effective Pain Relief
URL: http://bit.ly/CBD-Doses

Pg. 36: Cannabis as a Substitute for Opioid-Based Pain Medication: Patient Self-Report
URL: http://bit.ly/Opioid-Based

Pg. 37: MERRY JANE: What You Need to Know About Using Cannabis Suppositories
URL: http://bit.ly/CBD-Suppositories

Pg. 38: Cannabinoids & Your Vagina: the Science of Pleasure & Relief
URL: http://bit.ly/CBD-Vagina

Pg. 43: Medical Marijuana: The State of the Science
URL: http://bit.ly/MMJ-Science

Pg. 51: Kazmira: "How to Read Certificate of Analysis of Industrial Hemp Derived Products"
URL: http://bit.ly/CBD-COA

Pg. 52: JAMA: "Labeling Accuracy of Cannabidiol Extracts Sold Online"
URL: http://bit.ly/CBD-Labels

Pg. 64: Matador Network: No, CBD is not legal in all 50 states
URL: http://bit.ly/CBD-Legal

Back Cover: Centers for Disease Control and Prevention: Prevalence of Chronic Pain and High-Impact Chronic Pain Among Adults - United States, 2016
URL: http://bit.ly/CBD-Pain

THANK YOU

I want to give a special thank you to the father/daughter team over at testing facility G2 Analytical. The readers of this book will greatly benefit from your input and insight. G2 Analytical Can be reached through the following:

Veronica Griffin
P: (803) 415-9315
E: vgriffin@g2analytical.com
www.g2analytical.com

A special thank you goes out to friend Carly Goebel for her insights and dedication to helping others. If you want to connect with a social network that supports people who use Cannabis as an alternative therapy:

Carly Goebel | Founder & CEO, CannaCRPS Foundation
Direct: 310.486.4863
Carly@CannaCRPS.com | www.CannaCRPS.org

It should also be mentioned, NORML, the best-known organization to give consumers up-to-date information regarding cannabis and hemp laws. They should be one of your permanent bookmarks:

NORML and the NORML Foundation.
Direct: (202) 483-5500 | norml@norml.org
1100 H Street, NW
Suite 830
Washington, DC 20005
Membership/Donation: orders@norml.org
Legal Questions: legal@norml.org
https://norml.org

APPENDIX

CBD CHECKLIST

On the following page is a checklist for purchasing CBD oil and other products. It is not all-inclusive. The checklist gives you a basic guideline to follow when you have found a manufacturer that offers what you are searching for.

Product Label:

These are the essential elements you need to find on the label when you are ready to purchase CBD product. Review the list alongside the manufacturer's product label if you can. You will notice that there is an "X" indicator to let you know some items are required and some items are not. Eventually, we will get to a place in time where all these things will be required.

Company Website:

Follow this list when you are online looking at products you are considering buying. These are just some of the minimum things you should find and what you should look for.

Certificate of Analysis/Test Results:

Note: if you don't feel at ease reviewing lab tests, that's ok. Start where you are comfortable and grow from there. It's important that you do the 'Product Label' and 'Company Website' checklist. Following these two lists, you will purchase higher quality and safer product. Others will buy at random and risk buying bad quality medication.

You should at least review all the notes in red in this section.

Using this portion of the checklist should be pretty straight forward. Print any available test results and compare the two side by side as with the label.

NOTE: There is no independent analysis to support this next statement: only anecdotal evidence, experience, and knowledge of the industry.

More than one-third of the product on the market are trash. Here is the bottom line, and this is where you should draw your line. Lab test results should be "3rd party only." "Only Independent third-party lab test results should be used on what is "labeled and presented" for public consumption."

Checklist For Buying CBD OIL/Products

Description	Check list	Req'd	Notes
Product Label			
Name of Product		X	Do not purchase if missing product name.
Manufacturer/Distributer		X	Do not purchase if missing manufacturers name.
Batch Number			Most do not use batch numbers, yet. If they do, big plus for you.
Suggested Serving Size		X	
Servings Per Unit		X	
Volume		X	
Expiration Date		X	
Preservation Instructions			If not on label then on included user instructions.
Caution Statements			
QR Code/URL to COA on Product Packaging			If no URL to COA available on package, strongly consider not buying.
Company Website			
Website		X	Do not purchase if no company website.
Support Phone Number		X	
Duplicate Product Label		X	Should be the same as on product.
Download Test Results/COA		X	If they don't provide 3rd. party analysis that you can print, don't buy
Description of Product		X	
Certificate of Analysis (COA)/Test Results			
Name of Product		X	Do not purchase if missing product name.
Manufacturer		X	Do not purchase if missing manufacturers name.
Date Sample Received		X	
Dater Sample Tested		X	
Batch Number			
Test Results By 3rd Party		X	Perfect
Test Results By Company			SEE RED NOTES ON PREVIOUS PAGE
Is THC Content Less Than 0.03%		x	
Potency Analysis		X	
Heavy Metal Analysis			Not all tests include this but if they do, better for you.
Pesticide Analysis		X	If they don't test for pesticides don't purchase
Terpene Profiles			

ENDNOTES

Page ii

Doctors should be paid well for years of rigorous training to heal the human body. But federal data showed in 2015, 48% of physicians received some pharmaceutical payment. "It smells like doctors being bribed to sell narcotics, and that's very disturbing." - Dr. Andrew Kolodny, senior scientist at the Institute for Behavioral Health at the Heller School for Social Policy and Management at Brandeis University, and co-director of the Opioid Policy Research Collaborative.

Page 25

There is a variety of ways that CBD can be extracted from the hemp plant. If you really want to take this on, then you should learn more. This book is about the application of CBD products, so I did not spend a significant amount of time explaining. Here is one of the better resources to learn more about the extraction process.

How to Extract CBD – The Extraction Process & How CBD Oil is Made. URL: http://bit.ly/CBD-Extraction

FDA CONSUMER UPDATE
REGARDING
CBD PRODUCTS

Following is the Food and Drug Administration Consumer Update regarding CBD and products containing CBD. Before this update was posted, they simultaneously served 15 cannabis product manufacturers' notice to stop making unfounded claims on their products.

Boiled down, the FDA is telling companies you cannot put CBD in any food or dietary product and claim health benefits that cannot be substantiated by any medical or clinical corroboration. It's illegal to do so. They are watching; there are more snake-oil-salesman out there than you can imagine. But not all of them are.

Secondly, this update is the equivalent of a big-pharma drug company commercial telling you all of the destructive side effects that occur to your body while taking those REAL DRUGS. Now, in this case, there is no:

- Memory Loss
- Coughing Up Blood
- Suicidality
- Or Worse Death

Dr. Gregory Smith, the CEO of Red Pill Medical Inc., one of the companies noticed, makes a very valid point: the FDA's concerns regarding CBD are "a little misleading."

"The studies showing these problems were mainly done in animals who were given incredibly high doses of cannabis (if extrapolated to humans, no one under normal conditions could consume that much cannabis or CBD) that lead to liver issues. Also, the metabolism and absorption of CBD in the mice/rat model is very different than in humans," Smith says. "I have maintained that clinically, the safety profile of CBD is excellent, especially when compared to any prescription medication. This is not to say that consumers with medical problems taking prescription medications should not use CBD with caution."

I want to point out the only CBD "DRUG" approved by the FDA, had a dosage range of 500mgs to as high as 1,500mgs. That is an extreme amount of medical-grade CBD oil to ingest, multiple times a day. Yes, I can see why the concern for liver and stomach issues.

I speak for myself in this; the benefits outweigh the possible side effects they claim, especially for doses under 100mgs. There is much medical evidence to the contrary. But I will stand corrected if wrong. I will continue to use CBD for my pain relief.

REPRINTED FROM
THE
FDA WEBSITE

WHAT YOU NEED TO KNOW (AND WHAT WE'RE WORKING TO FIND OUT) ABOUT PRODUCTS CONTAINING CANNABIS OR CANNABIS-DERIVED COMPOUNDS, INCLUDING CBD

The FDA is working to answer questions about the science, safety, and quality of products containing cannabis and cannabis-derived compounds, particularly CBD.

> Content current as of:
> 11/25/2019
>
> Regulated Product(s):
> Animal & Veterinary
> Dietary Supplements
> Drugs
> Food & Beverages

- The FDA has approved only one CBD product, a prescription drug product to treat two rare, severe forms of epilepsy.
- It is currently illegal to market CBD by adding it to a food or labeling it as a dietary supplement.
- The FDA has seen only limited data about CBD safety and these data point to real risks that need to be considered before taking CBD for any reason.
- Some CBD products are being marketed with unproven medical claims and are of unknown quality.
- The FDA will continue to update the public as it learns more about CBD.

1. CBD has the potential to harm you, and harm can happen even before you become aware of it.
    - CBD can cause liver injury.
    - CBD can affect the metabolism of other drugs, causing serious side effects.
    - Use of CBD with alcohol or other Central Nervous System depressants increases the risk of sedation and drowsiness, which can lead to injuries.
2. CBD can cause side effects that you might notice. These side effects should improve when CBD is stopped or when the amount ingested is reduced.
    - Changes in alertness, most commonly experienced as somnolence (drowsiness or sleepiness).
    - Gastrointestinal distress, most commonly experienced as diarrhea and/or decreased appetite.
    - Changes in mood, most commonly experienced as irritability and agitation.
3. There are many important aspects about CBD that we just don't know, such as:
    - What happens if you take CBD daily for sustained periods of time?
    - What is the effect of CBD on the developing brain (such as children who take CBD)?
    - What are the effects of CBD on the developing fetus or breastfed newborn?
    - How does CBD interact with herbs and botanicals?
    - Does CBD cause male reproductive toxicity in humans, as has been reported in studies of animals?

You may have noticed that cannabidiol (CBD) seems to be available almost everywhere, and marketed as a variety of products including drugs, food, dietary supplements, cosmetics, and animal health products. Other than one prescription drug product to treat two rare, severe forms of epilepsy, the U.S. Food and Drug Administration (FDA) has not approved any other CBD products, and there is very limited available information about CBD, including about its effects on the body.

    7 Ways to Manage Pain with CBD

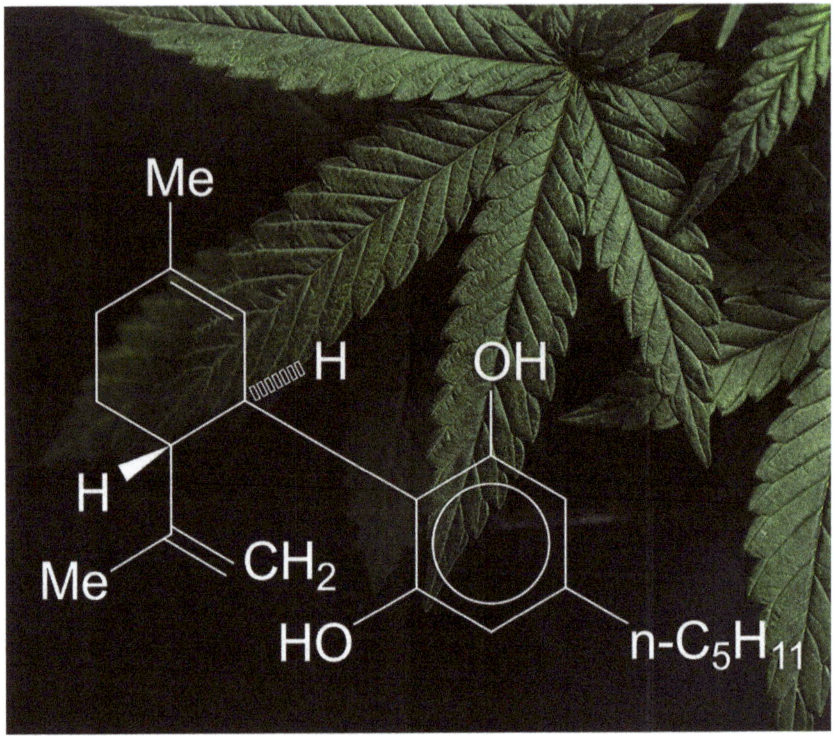

CBD chemical structure and marijuana leaves.

The FDA recognizes the significant public interest in cannabis and cannabis-derived compounds, particularly CBD. However, there are many unanswered questions about the science, safety, and quality of products containing CBD. The agency is working on answering these questions through ongoing efforts including feedback from a recent FDA hearing and information and data gathering through a public docket.

Despite the 2018 Farm Bill removing hemp — defined as cannabis and cannabis derivatives with very low concentrations (no more than 0.3% on a dry weight basis) of THC — from the definition of marijuana in the Controlled Substances Act, CBD products are still subject to the same laws and requirements as FDA-regulated products that contain any other substance.

The FDA is concerned that people may mistakenly believe that trying CBD "can't hurt." The agency wants to be clear that we have seen only limited data about CBD's safety and these data point to real risks that need to be considered. As part of the drug review and approval process for the prescription drug containing CBD, it was determined that the risks are outweighed by the benefits of the approved drug for the particular population for which it was intended. Consumer use of any CBD products should always be discussed with a healthcare provider. Consumers should be aware of the potential risks associated with using CBD products. Some of these can occur without your awareness, such as:

LIVER INJURY

During its review of the marketing application for Epidiolex — a purified form of CBD that the FDA approved in 2018 for use in the treatment of two rare and severe seizure disorders — the FDA identified certain safety risks, including the potential for liver injury. This serious risk can be managed when an FDA-approved CBD drug product is taken under medical supervision, but it is less clear how it might be managed when CBD is used far more widely, without medical supervision, and not in accordance with FDA-approved labeling. Although this risk was increased when taken with other drugs that impact the liver, signs of liver injury were seen also in patients not on those drugs. The occurrence of this liver injury was identified through blood tests, as is often the case with early problems with the liver. Liver injury was also seen in other studies of CBD in published literature. We are concerned about potential liver injury associated with CBD use that could go undetected if not monitored by a healthcare provider.

DRUG INTERACTIONS

Information from studies of the FDA-approved CBD drug Epidiolex show that there is a risk of CBD impacting other medicines you take – or that other medicines you take could impact the dose of CBD that can safely be used. Taking CBD with other medications may increase or decrease the effects of the other medications. This may lead to an increased chance of adverse effects from, or decreased effectiveness of, the other medications. Drug interactions were also seen in other studies of CBD in published literature. We are concerned about the potential safety of taking other medicines with CBD when not being monitored by a healthcare provider. In addition, there is limited research on the interactions between CBD products and herbs or botanicals in dietary supplements. Consumers should use caution when combining CBD products with herbs or dietary supplements.

MALE REPRODUCTIVE TOXICITY

Studies in laboratory animals showed male reproductive toxicity, including in the male offspring of CBD-treated pregnant females. The changes seen include decrease in testicular size, inhibition of sperm growth and development, and decreased circulating testosterone, among others. Because these findings were only seen in animals, it is not yet clear what these findings mean for human patients and the impact it could have on men (or the male children of pregnant women) who take CBD. For instance, these findings raise the concern that CBD could negatively affect a man's fertility. Further testing and evaluation are needed to better understand this potential risk.

In addition, CBD can be the cause of side effects that you might notice. These side effects should improve when CBD is stopped or when the amount ingested is reduced. This could include changes in alertness, most commonly experienced as somnolence (sleepiness), but this could also include insomnia; gastrointestinal distress, most commonly experienced as diarrhea and/or decreased appetite, but could also include abdominal pain or upset stomach; and changes in mood, most commonly experienced as irritability and agitation.

The FDA is actively working to learn more about the safety of CBD and CBD products, including the risks identified above and other topics, such as:

CUMULATIVE EXPOSURE

The cumulative exposure to CBD if people access it across a broad range of consumer products. For example, what happens if you eat food with CBD in it, use CBD-infused skin cream and take other CBD-based products on the same day? How much CBD is absorbed from your skin cream? What if you use these products daily for a week or a month?

SPECIAL POPULATIONS

The effects of CBD on other special populations (e.g., the elderly, children, adolescents, pregnant and lactating women).

CBD AND ANIMALS

The safety of CBD use in pets and other animals, including considerations of species, breed, or class and the safety of the resulting human food products (e.g., meat milk, or eggs) from food-producing species.

SOME CBD PRODUCTS ARE BEING MARKETED WITH UNPROVEN MEDICAL CLAIMS AND COULD BE PRODUCED WITH UNSAFE MANUFACTURING PRACTICES

Unlike the FDA-approved CBD drug product, unapproved CBD products, which could include unapproved drugs, cosmetics, foods, and products marketed as dietary supplements, have not been subject to FDA evaluation regarding whether they are effective to treat a particular disease or have other effects that may be claimed. In addition, they have not been evaluated by the FDA to determine what the proper dosage is, how they could interact with other drugs or foods, or whether they have dangerous side effects or other safety concerns.

Misleading, unproven, or false claims associated with CBD products may lead consumers to put off getting important medical care, such as proper diagnosis, treatment, and supportive care. For that reason, it's important to talk to your doctor about the best way to treat diseases or conditions with available FDA-approved treatment options.

In addition to safety risks and unproven claims, the quality of many CBD products may also be in question. The FDA is also concerned that a lack of appropriate processing controls and practices can put consumers at additional risks. For example, the agency has tested the chemical content of cannabinoid compounds in some of the products, and many were found to not contain the levels of CBD they claimed. We are also investigating reports of CBD potentially containing unsafe levels of contaminants (e.g., pesticides, heavy metals, THC).

CBD products are also being marketed for pets and other animals. The FDA has not approved CBD for any use in animals and the concerns regarding CBD products with unproven medical claims and of unknown quality equally apply to CBD products marketed for animals. The FDA recommends pet owners talk with their veterinarians about appropriate treatment options for their pets.

The FDA's top priority is to protect the public health. This priority includes making sure consumers know about products that put their health and safety at greatest risk, such as those claiming to prevent, diagnose, treat, mitigate, or cure serious diseases. For example, the agency has warned companies to stop selling CBD products they claim are intended to prevent, diagnose, treat, mitigate, or cure serious diseases such as

 7 Ways to Manage Pain with CBD

cancer, Alzheimer's disease, psychiatric disorders and diabetes. While we have focused on these types of products, we will continue to monitor the marketplace for any product that poses a risk to public health, including those with dangerous contaminants, those marketed to vulnerable populations, and products that otherwise put the public health at risk.

THE FDA IS CONTINUING TO EVALUATE THE REGULATORY FRAMEWORKS FOR PRODUCTS CONTAINING CANNABIS AND CANNABIS-DERIVED COMPOUNDS

The FDA continues to believe the drug approval process represents the best way to ensure that safe and effective new medicines, including any drugs derived from cannabis, are available to patients in need of appropriate medical therapy. The agency is committed to supporting the development of new drugs, including cannabis and cannabis-derived drugs, through the investigational new drug and drug approval process.

We are aware that there may be some products on the market that add CBD to a food or label CBD as a dietary supplement. Under federal law, it is illegal to market CBD this way.

The FDA is evaluating the regulatory frameworks that apply to certain cannabis-derived products that are intended for non-drug uses, including whether and/or how the FDA might consider updating its regulations, as well as whether potential legislation might be appropriate. The information we have underscores the need for further study and high quality, scientific information about the safety and potential uses of CBD.

The FDA is committed to setting sound, science-based policy. The FDA is raising these safety, marketing, and labeling concerns because we want you to know what we know. We encourage consumers to think carefully before exposing themselves, their family, or their pets, to any product, especially products like CBD, which may have potential risks, be of unknown quality, and have unproven benefits.

Our Consumer Update includes a practical summary of what we know to date. As we learn more, our goal is to update you with the information you need to make informed choices about CBD products. Also, as the regulatory pathways are clarified we will take care to inform all stakeholders as quickly as possible.

U.S. Food & Drug Administration References

This article

FDA: What You Need to Know (And What We're Working to Find Out) About Products Containing Cannabis or Cannabis-derived Compounds, Including CBD.

Link: http://bit.ly/fda-warning

Article Image: U.S. Food & Drug Administration, CBD chemical structure and marijuana leaves. 2019, Retrieved from URL: https://www.fda.gov/files/cbd-chemical-structure-marijuana-leaves-900x900.jpg

FDA cannabis/food regulation article (Recommended read)

FDA: FDA Regulation of Cannabis and Cannabis-Derived Products, Including Cannabidiol (CBD)

Link: http://bit.ly/fda-cannabis-regs

Pg. 76: Cannabis Business Times: FDA Warns of CBD Use and Marketing, Companies Respond: Dr. Gregory Smith response to FDA warning letter.

URL: http://bit.ly/RedPillMed

DISCLAIMER

This book details the author's personal experiences with and opinions about managing pain symptoms with the use of CBD also known as cannabidiol from the hemp plant. The author is not a [or your] healthcare provider.

The author and publisher are providing this book and its contents on an "as is" basis and make no representations or warranties of any kind with respect to this book or its contents. The author and publisher disclaim all such representations and warranties, including for example warranties of merchantability and healthcare for a particular purpose. In addition, the author and publisher do not represent or warrant that the information accessible via this book is accurate, complete or current.

THESE STATEMENTS HAVE NOT BEEN EVALUATED BY THE FOOD AND DRUG ADMINISTRATION. THIS BOOK IS NOT INTENDED TO DIAGNOSE, TREAT, CURE , OR PREVENT ANY DISEASE. PLEASE CONSULT WITH YOUR OWN PHYSICIAN OR HEALTHCARE SPECIALIST REGARDING THE SUGGESTIONS AND RECOMMENDATIONS MADE IN THIS BOOK.

Except as specifically stated in this book, neither the author or publisher, nor any authors, contributors, or other representatives will be liable for damages arising out of or in connection with the use of this book. This is a comprehensive limitation of liability that applies to all damages of any kind, including (without limitation) compensatory; direct, indirect or consequential damages; loss of data, income or profit; loss of or damage to property and claims of third parties.

You understand that this book is not intended as a substitute for consultation with a licensed healthcare practitioner, such as your physician. Before you begin any healthcare program, or change your lifestyle in any way, you will consult your physician or another licensed healthcare practitioner to ensure that you are in good health and that the examples contained in this book will not harm you.

This book provides content related to physical health issues. As such, use of this book implies your acceptance of this disclaimer.

OUR AUTHOR

DAVID SCHROEDER

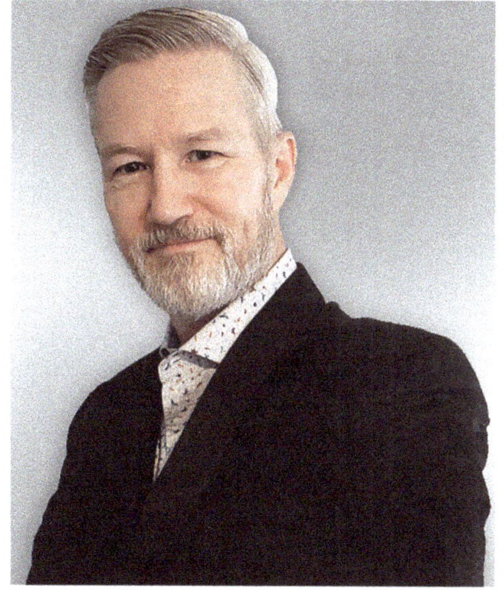

Throughout my life, I've suffered and lived with all types of injuries. In my youth, it was riding BMX bikes flying off of jumps and occasionally losing the front wheel, skateboarding was becoming a new fad before all the high flying tricks that we have today, and of course, we didn't wear helmets back in the day and crashing was the norm.

In my late teens and early adulthood, I was heavily into martial arts and agonized over crazy backaches and a myriad of other injuries. My favorite was sparring, I loved to clash, but I often got my butt kicked.

When I got into my late 20's and early 30's it was about rollerblading and mountain biking. I even participated in 3-day long trips, peddling a hundred miles a day. I was no stranger to pain or injury.

When I hit 40, because of the amount of time spent behind a computer, I experienced a whole new level of aches and pains.

I've used many types of topicals over the years, such as Bengay, Tiger Balm, Icy Hot, Bio-Freeze, and others. Some worked, some didn't. But one important factor, they weren't anti-inflammatory in nature.

Now I look back over the years, and I see that they did provide some minor relief! But only minor relief. Yes, I will agree, they did provide some heat to the local area where applied. But they didn't reduce inflammation.

It has only been three years (2016) since I discovered the use of CBD in topicals. I recognized almost immediate relief upon use, and then shortly thereafter, I began to explore other ways of getting pain relief using CBD. From my explorations we have this beautiful book, 7 Way To Manage Pain With CBD.

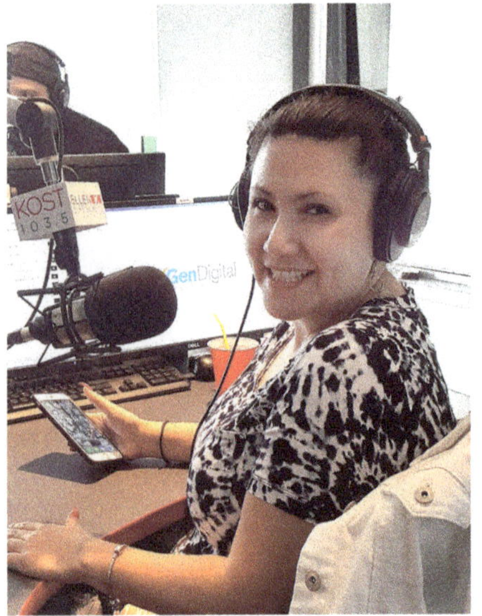

JESSICA RIVAS

I also want to give a very special thank you to a couple of contributors. The first, Jessica Rivas. My best friend, my confidante, my life partner, my right and left hand. Her guidance, counsel, and motivation help keep on course. Without her, I'm only half a person.

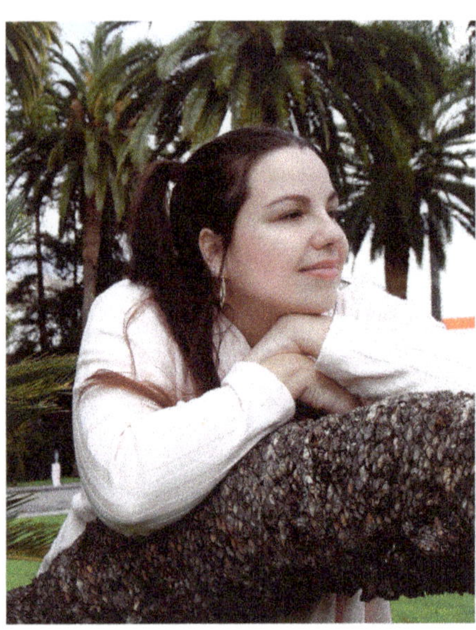

ALIA PARISE

And to Alia Parise. She gave my baby life. Yea I could have done the graphics and the book layout, but it would have been old school fuddy-duddy, boring stuff. Alia, she brought personality, life, love of her craft, and excellence and made this book fun.